# Forever Slim

# Forever Slim

*Mary Bray, M.A.*

Writers Club Press
San Jose  New York  Lincoln  Shanghai

**Forever Slim**

All Rights Reserved © 2001 by Mary Bray

Writers Club Press
an imprint of iUniverse, Inc.

For information address:
iUniverse, Inc.
5220 S. 16th St., Suite 200
Lincoln, NE 68512
www.iuniverse.com

ISBN: 0-595-14815-8

Printed in the United States of America

# *Contents*

# *INTRODUCTION*

FOREVER THIN is a *What to do* and *How to do* step by step guide to reaching your ideal weight. There is only one requirement and that is...that you don't go on any kind of a diet! That has never worked and never will.

This guide is what you have waited for, a fool proof surety that it will work for you **when you do it** step by step. This book is really about learning what to do to create for **you** your ideal weight once and for all. This is a learning process, and once you have learned it, you can stay with your ideal body forever. Actually it's not even much to do about food!

You will discover with pleasure **your own resources** (that you never thought possible), will make it work, revealing to yourself **your own power** through self direction and auto suggestion while deeply relaxed and inspired to learn more about your creativity, and open doors to all you desire that is possible for you.

My fat story

I started to notice, when I was in high school, that I was not like the other girls. I weighted about 40 pounds more than all the rest of the girls. I was in a program it was called Donaldsons-Teenboard, and in this program one person was represented from every high school. I was 16 years old and the representatives, one from each high school, told other class maids about events that were happening at Donaldsons in the way of fashion shows and learning how to be graceful for young girls. I also worked at Donaldsons. Of course that was good for the store, because I brought in my high school friends to Donaldsons to buy clothes. But it was like you were recognized as having a special job. Of course it was really only fashionable beautiful girls, who were chosen to be on this particular teenboard. Now it wasn't the best teenboard in the city. The best teenboard was at Dayton's, where the girls were more beautiful. I noticed that, when we were trying on our clothes, that we would wear as representatives of the high school, that I had to order special size—and the size was 16.

In a few months, when we change the season and new clothes had to be ordered, I had to order a size 18. I remembered being so embarassed, and somehow I didn't make the connection, that I was just plain fat. And worse than that I had no idea how to change. Everybody said to me: "Oh Mary you are such a wonderful personality, it doesn't matter what you weigh". That's what they thought! Mary you aren't fat, you just have big bones.

I had a boyfriend, when I began to notice, that the top guys, the football players, the athletes, the presidents of the students council, that caliber of young men, weren't choosing me to go to the homecoming dance, or to go to the spring formal, and this was absolutely crushing. I didn't know if it was because I was fat, or because I was just not attractive. I always ended up going to the dance, but I ended up going as the last choice. And so I learned over the years to **accept second best**, because of course, that's what I thought I was capable of and therefore all that I deserved. I had a special blow, and that was when my first love, who didn't care if I was fat or thin, or so he said, chose another girl, to ask to his senior prom, and the girl was very small, 98 pounds soaking wet, I'm sure and not more. All of a sudden I made the association, that I was going to be fat, and second best. I had no idea how to lose the weight, I had no idea what that meant, that I was eating too much and of course when I felt insecure, I substituted food for comfort. And when all boys and girls got together at the Drive-In and they went of in each other's cars, I sat in the Drive-In and ate one or two hamburgers and at least frenchfries and malt, and never noticed that the other girls only drank a coke or a lemonade.

Being fat predicted a lot of my behavior. To this very day, I have sometimes catched myself as I slip into old thoughts of believing I'm still overweight and unattractive. My memory goes back to days at the beach noticing the boys paying attention to other girls who were thin, and suffering bigtime because I had no idea how to change to be the person I really felt inside. I had so many girl friends, and I heard over and over their stories of which boy they should go out with, and I suffered with no dates. No strong young men picked me up at the beach and tossed me in the water in fun and frolick.

So I ate to heal my wounds and spent a lot of time going out to eat with girlfriends. And this became my identity. At 17 years old Mary is fat—but she has a personality. She is fun…fat and happy. Of course no one but my best friend Janice knew how I suffered. I just didn't understand why my legs were twice the size of hers.

My greatest dream at the time was to be a flight attendant and so I wrote to Dallas Texas with Braniff airlines, and I said: "What do I have to do to become an airline hostess". The first thing they said was: "You can't weigh more than a 130 pounds". Well I always weighed 160 or more. I thought to myself, I'm going to lose this weight. I went to the doctor, told the doctor I wanted to lose weight, and he gave me medicine to lose weight, to curb my appetite. Well I took this medicine and it was like I was flying, because of course it was an amphetamine. And so I would take the medicine and never had any interest in eating, but thought I was going crazy. I accomplished many things in a day, because I was totally hyperactive, and then I was so tired at the end of the day and also in the morning, that I had to give up the pills. And when I gave up the pills, I ate more than ever!

Well I had another idea, I thought, there is another way, that food comes out. So I'll take a few exlax or a diuretic. So I took exlax and a diuretic and continued eating what I thought was normal. I never told anybody about that. Threee days before I went to the interview, I sat on the toilet all the way to Dallas, and for the next two days, while I waited for my interview to take place. I starved, didn't eat anything, because I thought, whatever I ate would make me fat. I went to the interview and they said: "We like your application, and it's possible for you to work for us, but you have to lose 13 pounds".

I thought I'm going to do it what ever it takes. So I continued with my program of amphetamines and exlax and made the weighing three weeks later at 130 pounds exactly. I didn't even drink coffee that morning or any water, just by chance, that I wouldn't make it.

Naturally after I made the weighing and got the job, I resumed my old habits.

In the first three months of flying with Braniff-Airlines, we had to weigh in once a month. And I thought, well it's a little bit over it can't really hurt, because I already had the job. When the chief hostess said to me: "Mary, I see that you are 7 pounds overweight. We will have to ground you, until you lose the weight, without pay.

Well, the story goes on…after each baby (3) I seemed to have an extra 10 or 20 pounds, and I was still in the habit of eating with the belief that celebrating means eating and the more one eats, the more fun one has, and everyone feels full and satisfied, and to me that meant it was a good day. If my three sons ate a lot, they were also happy, and that meant I was a good mother. The better it tasted, the more I ate. After all more is better, right?

Every new diet that came out on the market, I tried. Dr. Stillmans, Adkins, drinking what tasted like liquid chalk, and sometimes I lost weight, but when stress or problems came up, I went back to overeating all the foods that I learned gave me pleasure. I really didn't know what else to do.

I heard about so called fat farms and dreamed about going to one to have someone magically cure me and make me thin. I felt trapped in my body, a wall of fat preventing me from enjoying life. I stood between the real world of pleasure and my illusion that food was my refuge. I went to school and worked in a clinic there, I began to realize in my early 40s that as I was teaching others how to get well and thin and how to stop hurting physically and mentally, I had not shown myself the delight of being at my ideal weight. And like all decisions happen, eventually one day I decided **to ask for help.**

I went that day in the hospital where I was working to Dr. David Axelrad, my colleague for whom I would trust my life. I had seen him heal others as if by magic. He also had one time healed himself after a near tragic auto accident, where he had such a severe head injury that one cough or sneeze or movement could cause the delicate tissues in his brain, and in his head to burst causing instant death.

Being a psychiatrist, he knew exactly the severity of the situation, and he began to heal himself with his own thinking and self hypnosis. He studied the great works of Dr. Milton Erickson, also a Psychiatrist and known as the Father of Hypnosis. David learned and acted on every sentence, every skill, every tool that Dr. Erickson offered. As he fully recovered, he made the decision to show others how to **self direct their lives,** so as to heal themselves and make intended changes, without suffering pain or the side effects of medication.

One of the side effects of certain kinds of pain medication is an increased appetite with increased weight gain.

So I went to him and all I said was: "David, I don't want to be overweight anymore". I was at the time 165 pounds. "I'm trying to show others how to lose weight and conquer their pain, and I'm not doing what I want for myself, and what I have wanted for 30 YEARS". He stopped what he was doing and said: "So you are ready to lose weight". I said: "Yes, that is what I want more than anything in the whole world. I've suffered enough. Do you think you can help *even me*?". He smiled and said: "Have you got 20 minutes?". I said: "Yes, why?". He said: "Come into my office and sit down". He suggested I deeply relax and proceeded to offer me the same imagination, the same process that I knew only so well, because it was so successful with all the patients, **I just hadn't done it myself** yet, and after that session I left the office and went to a dinner party. I wasn't sure why I was crying on the way to the party, but I felt like some kind of relief going on inside myself. Later I realized he took me in his office at that moment because I was READY to shed all that weight, I had made the decision, and I had a hearts **desire** to be free from that wall of fat. Behind that wall was a beautiful woman on the inside—imprisoned by old habits of eating. Hunger wasn't even a consideration for me. I didn't wait until I was hungry to eat. I ate from frustration, boredom and being unsatisfied with myself. It seemed to give comfort…or so I thought. You know.

In the biofeedback session, I focused on my dream to be thin and trusted him unconditionally. In my imagination I saw myself slim and beautiful, really beautiful, running in white shorts, and a white t-shirt, my hair blowing in the wind. I saw myself weighing 128 pounds, where before I had never even **thought** about that being a possibility. I could feel my movement, like I was flowing, and my face was radiant. My tears were partly release and relief, and partly tears of joy. I am crying now, as I remember it, because my image became a reality and that's the reason for this book, because it is my hearts desire to make your life a little lighter, or a lot lighter **now** and to begin this very day.

I went to the dinner party, and of course, there was so much food, and as I moved toward the table, I know I had made a change, I was just no longer interested in a table full of food, because I had a kind of full feeling in my own self. I know there was no stopping me to become the person I always wanted to be. Six months later I weighed 40 pounds less.

At age 46 I bought my first bikini, a black one. Black makes one look smaller, right? This is the power of imagination, believing in the possibility, and trusting your thoughts to put you in the physical state of TAKING ACTION.

Every Action has an equal and opposite reaction.

So in the following chapters of this book, you will find all the steps you need on how to take your own action. I think you must be ready, or getting ready to make the decision to lose the amount of weight you desire, or at least you are curious about your own possibilities.

So let's get started. I'm excited for the opportunity to pass on to you all that I know about LOSING WEIGHT and keeping it off forever!

# CHAPTER 1

## *Everything begins with a thought or an idea*

The reality of thoughts and the power they have can create and change the lives of all persons willing to listen and be aware of their own self desires and the creative power they have within themselves. I truly believe every person in the world wants and needs to be fulfilled to meet their needs and find pleasure. At least that's how it begins and it's the way nature works, in so far as…all persons and animals are equipped with survival instincts, and the basic needs for survival which are food, warmth and love. What a child learns quickly from bonding with the mother that she will respond to those needs when the baby cries, and also that the baby will not stop crying until these needs are met. Now humans have this distinct characteristic that no other animal has…and that is the ability to think and reason. Soon follows the ability to choose. It's not so very long before the child learns to think the following:

1. If my mother is not near me, I must wait for food
2. If my mother is not near me, there will be no food
3. If my mother is not near me, or she goes away, the child develops a fear that she may never come back, and therefore the child will not survive (Jean Piaget, "Child Psychology, Egocentric patterns of thinking ages 2-5"). This is the reason why children cry when mother leaves. A

child can also feel when the mother is emotionally tense, for sometimes the mother can project her tension or anger on to the child and the child response is fear, or an equivalent anxious feeling. It can be a warning signal to the child that he or she is not safe. As the child grows older the mother may become displeased with the child and a child has no way of understanding the meaning of this behavior, but at some level the child learns if he or she pleases the mother there is less concern for

1. getting their needs met in a comfortable environment
2. more surety that the mother will be there to feed them.

At the same time a child learns that he or she is rewarded with love and praise for being "a good boy" or a "good girl" especially at meal time when a sufficient amount of food has been consumed. Example: "You are such a big boy" or "What a nice big girl" and now the child's need for love becomes a pattern over and over at the dining table. Good feelings are being combined with the amount of food eaten...or eating to please mother.

At the same time, a child learns that when he or she **pleases the parents**, the child will receive the needs required for survival, and that allows the child to be fulfilled. The mother may even brag about how much the child has eaten, and how much milk he or she drank, and in such a way that the mother also feels fulfilled by satisfying the child's needs, because that indicates in part that she is also a good mother. "Are they getting enough milk, are they getting enough food. Moms want to do their best! More is better, right?

According to Milton Erickson "Patterns of Behavior 1" these patterns of behavior are followed as a child learns to think and associate with what brings pleasure and what brings pain. **All persons** will go to great lengths to gain pleasure and fulfillment, and even greater lengths to avoid pain. Early in life we all learn that pleasing the person who feeds us brings rewards of the pleasure of love and fulfillment and the notion that we are good!

At the same time, children can also internalize a not good feeling within their identity if they for instance, don't eat all the food provided for them at the time it is provided, even if the child is **not hungry**. So the child learns to eat all that is provided, hungry or not, because that means he or she will receive love and or indications of approval. Of course, well meaning parents have the positive intention of inspiring their child to be healthy and growing, and so many times the child is forced to eat more than they need, and only then are they able to be rewarded with dessert. Now all the while as the child's **thinking patterns are developing, so are the behavior patterns,** and here is where eating patterns and behaviors are developed.

It is only beginning at the age of 12 that a youngster can think from two sides, meaning their own point of view, and the point of view of another person, but even then when a twelve or thirteen year old recognizes their own thoughts and ideas, they are not in many cases able to say **"no"** to their parents. And consider this notion at the eating table. The young person acknowledges what they personally like and dislike, and just exactly how much food he or she wants and needs to eat, however in order to please the parents, they must do as directed or the consequence can have the potential of resulting in a painful or emotionally negative situation, which indicates the young person is not good; and even worse…not deserving love, which can be the **child's interpretation.**

Such is the case of a child for example not eating everything on his provided plate. Actually he can be subject to some form of punishment such as not being able to play if the entire meal is not eaten, or even sent to their room. The parents are of course well meaning and doing the best they know how, as far as fulfilling their obligation as responsible parents raising children. Here is where eating patterns and habits begin and are repeated for years until the child grows up and leaves home, and many times on into the next generation where the process continues. Since most discussions in the family take place around the dining table, it can be a time also of feelings and emotions being emitted, judgments made and punishment administered. Some of you may have the experience of being reprimanded at the dinner table, and as a result haven't felt like eating at all, and the situation could become worsened if no eating took place. To clean the plate then could be the redeeming effort, just to be able to leave the scene.

Historically the evidence of a prospering family is the abundance of food on the table, and it is a well known fact that throwing away or leaving food on one's plate could be anything from not adhering to family rules, to a mortal sin. As the saying goes, one must finish all the food that is provided because "What about the starving children in Africa?", or someplace where a hungry child would gladly send it. While these kinds of issues make no sense to a child at all, he or she can easily learn to feel guilty for not complying with the notions of the parents whom the child is always trying to please.

A child thinks everything the parents say and do is the way all of life is until one day they begin to have thoughts and ideas of their own, and begin to realize they can think for themselves and that they can either do what they want or they can respond to someone else's plan, but to change their direction to fulfill their self desires, can be a painful change. Not being accepted can hurt a lot! I have seen many people who still apologize to perfect strangers, waiters and waitresses, who couldn't care less what they ate, because they still have a feeling of guilt for not eating all the food on their plate even if they are full. **Habits and messages are all recorded in the brain,** and these thoughts messages and habits rule our lives, and for some persons for years and years, without even thinking about changing these habits or realizing we can.

But .... the wonderful asset that human beings have over all other animals is the **power to control and change their own thinking. The power of choice making.** Now many persons think and would like to change others rather than their own habits that are no longer useful, and I believe it's really the point that many people do not realize the pleasure they can exercise by governing their own **choice** over themselves. Thoughts are things. They are conceived in the mind and they travel through time and space affecting all that they touch. We can say that thoughts are the buildings blocks of our experience. The world that we see is the one that we have created with our thoughts. We think a thought, we attach a feeling to it, and a circumstance in our life is attracted to it. If we want to see how we arrived, where we are in life, we need only to trace our experience back to our thoughts, patterns and choices.

Remember as you developed and grew up as a child, not only did you receive messages from mothers and fathers and family members, but as you grew up, you learned what to think about yourself through friends, where what others thought about you was the major consideration. "What will others think of me?" A child then doesn't realize self control as a possibility as their identity is the mirror image they have of themselves from others. An interesting way overeating can occur during these stages is when a youngster has hurt feelings from a playmate or someone who shames the child or punishes such as a child receiving punishment in school.

The child and adults as well, will eat to receive the same fulfillment they received when they needed food or warmth or love in the past. And as the years go by this repeated behavior can be a cause for resorting to eating to meet other needs, to ease frustration, or meet the need of receiving love. It's a well known fact that rewards are given through cookies, sweets and treats that could have been replaced with a **hug.**

When we are aware of these patterns of behavior, we can control and regulate them and for this reason the topic of thinking is the first chapter in this book. We can make the choice to control and direct our thinking through **awareness** and then change to meet our new **identity, our desired self.**

As you look at all the cars driving by on the highway, or the rush hour traffic, what do you think is driving those cars? THOUGHTS. That's what is driving them. Someone woke up that morning and had a thought: "Let's go to the mountains today" or "Today I must fix my car" or "I need to go and see my friend"…each car is being led by a thought.

Everything we see in fact is a result of thought. "Your body is a result of thoughts, in a form you can see" said "Jonathan Livingston Seagull" by Richard Bach. This is easy to understand if we use a house as an example. Every house has been built only after an idea has given birth. Can you imagine a house being built before someone had a thought to construct it? Houses always come from the design that has been created by a thought. The opposite is never true. In the same way, our thoughts create the design for our circumstances. We are all born into a certain set of circumstances in a specific culture and a specific family.

To become aware that we have the capability to design, alter, and change our history is the first step in realizing it is our thoughts that create our reality. If you have a calm mind, you have a relaxed body. Every thought is a cause set in motion and our behavior follows what we choose to become.

If there is any stress, resistance, or limiting beliefs in your mind, it will show evidence in your body. In other words, it is only your mind or your thinking that prevents you from being reaching your ideal weight, and not your body. Isn't that a comforting message? You don't even have to believe it…yet, and as you continue reading with a faith that you are in control of your thoughts you are already on the path to living your desire to reach your ideal self exactly as you think and imagine yourself to be.

If we want to change your circumstances, we must change the way we think. We cannot allow ourselves only idle thought because there is no such thing. We can think rather of every thought as a seed. What we plant in our mental garden will grow. This is how the mind works!

> Sow a thought, reap an idea
> Sow an idea, reap an action
> Sow an action, reap a habit
> Sow a habit, reap a character
> Sow a character, reap a purpose
> Sow a purpose, reap a destiny

**Everything begins with a thought or an idea.**

To demonstrate the relationship between thoughts and the body, I often offer the following exercise in seminars: I ask a strong bodied person in the group to stretch out his or her arms while thinking of a stressful situation in life. Then I ask the person to keep their arms outstretched while I try to press them down while continuing to think about their own stressful situation. I have tested this hundreds of times, and I was able to press their arms down easily even though they tried in vain to hold them outstretched. Then I asked them to think about a wonderful vacation that they enjoyed and felt fulfilled. This time the arm becomes so strong that I could hardly move them. Try this simple exercise.

Mental stress weakens the physical body, and mental ease strengthens it. Our bodies are a mirror of our thoughts. Try this simple experiment with a partner, and while holding your arms outstretched, think about your present stressful situation about being overweight. You may see yourself fat, and how this brings you discomfort…about the way you look or feel, the discomfort of how you move, or feel your oversized clothes becoming tight, and tell yourself, I don't like how my body feels and looks. When you are in the state of thinking about your condition of having excess weight, nod your head and your partner can then proceed to lower both arms at once by pressing down.

Next, think about a time when you felt wonderful about your body, how you moved and how you looked, and the pleasure and enjoyment you experienced with yourself or another person or persons. It's O.K. to go back a long time to a time you may have almost forgotten and stretch out your arms reliving the experience in your mind. Nod your head again and your partner can again attempt to press your arms down. Just notice the difference and play with this exercise.

The mind and the body absolutely works together.

One day while enroute to my office on the train there was a delay in the train schedule. I found myself standing in the dismal cold crowded station with hundreds of others who seemed to be disgruntled over the situation of being late to their destinations, when I caught the eye of a small elderly man with a cain. In the midst of all the other people he seemed to have a light energy about him, so I continued observing him with this light hearted attitude as he was walking up and down the platform with a spring in his walk eventhough he had a limp. He noticed I was looking at him and he returned my observation with a smile. While the mechanics were adjusting the difficulty of the train, others were shifting their feet hunched over waiting in the cold with an aura of impatience. I decided to investigate what kind of a thought process was going on in this man's mind and so I moved closer to him and greeted him with a friendly smile and said something trivial like "It's too bad the train was late". I could barely understand his dialect, but he said he was using this time to walk up and down the platform to exercise his legs because if he sits too long on the train they become stiff, and when he said it he had a twinkle in his eye. His light hearted energy sparked mine and I instantly changed my state of chilled impatience to match this man's energy. My thoughts instantly changed, it was like a chain reaction, and as I saw this man turning a problem into an opportunity, I felt grateful to him for bringing me back to knowing I could also change my thoughts.

I didn't sit near him the rest of the journey but when I reached my destination I found him, gave him my best sparkle in my eye and told him to have a good day. The fact that the train was late became irrelevant in my thinking and after I thought about the reality of thoughts and the power they have to create and to change the world around us. By the time we see a circumstance, we are seeing the effect of a series of events that began with a thought long ago. Any change in circumstances is due only to a change in the way we think. Your thoughts are the key to your freedom. The power to change your destiny is in your hands. Your thinking can overcome all doubts for you who know the miracle of thought and the miracle of choices know the secret of life and can change your world.

As the train went off in the distance, I saw the man waving…twinkling until the train was out of sight.

# Chapter 2

## *Desire: Wishes and Dreams*

Just as our thoughts are the windows to our mind, we can also say our imagination is the workshop. And it is desire to act on our thoughts that creates the motion and the movement toward our goals and outcomes.

Our thoughts give us an indication and a glimpse even if it is ever so faint at first,…of possibilities that before a certain thought had never occurred to us before.

While I was working in a hospital in Houston Texas, I was teaching and training Biofeedback and the benefits of deep relaxation in a trance state to the patients who were there for various reasons related recovering from chronic pain. I was also encouraging some persons with chronic back pain to lose weight so as to create less strain on their back. Some of them had gained too much weight as a result of being inactive. Sometimes depression became a factor which can cause eating more amounts of food than needed just for seeking comfort in a time of physical impairment. I use this example to show you how a thought can jump into our mind sometimes when we least expect it. In this case, a patient and myself were entering a deep state of relaxation, and I was particularly training the skills of visual imagery. There was a calendar reminding me of my travels in Switzerland hanging on the wall in the biofeedbackroom and I fondly looked at it from time to time as I looked forward to returning there in the months to come. On this particular month there was a picture of a red cable car against a mountain background in the alps, and I found I was noticing the red cable car myself as I was leading my patient into visually imagining a pleasant surrounding where he had been before that was comfortable and relaxing while he was going into a deep relaxation. All of a sudden a thought came into my mind about the beauty I was seeing on the calendar. I imagined a picture of myself in Switzerland walking in the mountains of the alps with patients walking with me as they were recovering in the beauty of nature, breathing the fresh mountain air and getting well. Then I became excited and interested in my thought, and when I just allowed the thoughts to come into my head, I began to wonder if this could really be a possibility. In the following weeks my mind went back to this image and a feeling or an excitement caused me to have fun thinking about it. The more I thought about it, the more interesting it became. I went to sleep dreaming about it and many times woke up with this picture in my mind. I began to talk about it with friends I respected and sometimes they encouraged me. The next time I went to Switzerland I began trying to meet people who would be interested in my story and one day I took the risk. I moved to Switzerland and got a job in a souvenir shop selling and engraving Swiss Army knives. I went on to teach English, but I always took every step I could think of to pursue my dream. Three years later, my first 2 clients arrived in Switzerland from USA, and we walked in the mountains and breathed the fresh air while they recovered from their addictions, and flew back to the states. The dream, followed by my untention became my life work, my purpose, my destiny.

So you see, as I have told this true story, I replicate this process below.

                Thought
                     Idea
                       Imagination
                      Feeling
                       Desire
                            Persistence
                           Outcome state
                            Decision
                                Physical Action

The same diagram applies to weight loss.

Thought—Others are thin, why not me?
Idea—I am interested in being thin.
Feeling—Fear it is not possible
Desire—All my life I've wanted to be thin
Feeling—Fear it's not possible
Persistence—Ask for help
Focus—On desire, to lose weight
Imagination—Deep trance with visualization
Outcome—I will lose 40 pounds
State—Excitement about the possibility
Decision—I will never be fat again
Physical State—Taking action every day
Picture—I saw myself thin
Speaking—I told myself there is no going back
Feeling—Proud of my action and decision
Success

Here are the exact steps for you to follow.
You are already here:

1. Know your outcome
2. Put it to your imagination
3. Make a decision
4. Learn to believe in the possibility through your small steps forward
5. What do you value? What do you really want?
6. Planning
7. Rolemodeling
8. Managing your state inside and out, allowing you feelings of being convinced
9. "I can do this". That is you new belief about yourself!

"See it, Do it, Be it!"

When you think about how much you will enjoy being your desired self, and allow your thoughts to run wild about how this will positively effect your life …. What happens? Do you recognize and see it as a possibility for a while, and then get interrupted by thoughts that it is not possible? Do you get distracted, do you put it off?

What has to happen for you to stand up in the morning with a compelling desire to react and reach your goal every day of becoming exactly the body size you want? What conditions have to happen for you to be unstoppable, and for you to be highly motivated…so that you flow through the day totally successful toward the desired amount of weight you want to lose? Let's try an experiment here with which is a convenient short cut method of finding out how you program and run your brain.

You already have all the resources you need inside your brain to become your desired wheight, and in this chapter you are going to learn how to direct your own resources. Why? So you can have what you want. We are not going to focus on your being fat, because if we focus on that we wouldn't be focusing on a solution, would we? Thinking about being fat has never made you thin before, has it? In fact, the reverse happens, when you think about your present overweight condition you only become demotivated, down, and a little depressed, right? In fact it closes the doors to the possibility of being thin, doesn't it? Try it once. Think about all the attempts you've tried before to become thin and failed. Think about how you were going to try to lose weight and ended up getting fatter. Think about how your clothes don't fit and the ones that are hanging in the closet that you can't wear that were so expensive.Think about others telling you to lose weight. Think of yourself telling yourself: "You've got to start a diet". See yourself feeling out of control...............STOPPPPPPP !!!!

Now, notice how you feel. Do you feel motivated or have a desire to be thin now? Do you feel excited at the possibility of losing all the weight you desire? NO! You have shut down the possibility with your **thinking about the problem** and focusing on it, haven't you? What if I were to tell you that you have also the resources within yourself to change this goom doom thinking to positive stimulating burning desire to become thin, a new you...stunning in appearance and vital with flowing lean movement? (Sounds like a commercial, right)?

*"Nothing has any power over you than that which you give it through your thoughts."* (Antony Robbins, "Unlimited Power").

We represent our negative emotions and positive emotions with our senses seeing, hearing, touching, smelling, feeling. While thinking and focusing on the issues in your life as a result of being overweight, notice if you formed a picture in your mind while thinking about your fat condition. Did you see yourself fat? Go back and do it again. Notice if you had a feeling connected with being overweight, like bulky or bloated or guilty or frustrated. Did you say anything to yourself like: "You shouldn't have eaten so much" or "I should go on a diet"? Just notice this way you have of representing and make a written note. At least take a moment to think about it.

Now remember a time in your life when you first fell in love, and you were flirting. (It's great to think about it, isn't it?) Take some time with this before you move on because it can show you the power of your own resources. Can you picture yourself with your loved one? Even if you are no longer with this person, you can still recall the wonder of the experience, can't you? Were there any special smells involved or feelings like "If this is not heaven it's a close second"? Feelings of warmth, touch, and eyes sparkling .... Did you say anything to yourself or have a conversation? You are learning how your brain works, and it's important because you can reflect on your past experiences where you felt your zest and desire for life and transfer that to your desired goal of weight loss by understanding how you think in the way that you respond with motivation and desire.

OK Let's try another one.
Remember a time when you were absolutely successful at something? Anything. For example you completed a project, you passed a test, you got the job you wanted. Now see everything you saw when you were so successful, who was there, where were you, and what did people say about your success and what did you tell yourself? Were you proud, excited, estatic? And how did that feel? Where did you feel it in your body? In your stomach? Butterflies in your stomach, a feeling of fullness? Yeah? OK, now you are getting the idea. If you are having difficulty with this, stop right now and go back to the beginning of this chapter until you get yourself to the feeling of fullness from your

success. As you remember your success you will have no difficulty learning how to experience them again.

OK here's the next step.

While you're experiencing your success scene, run it on a movie screen as if it were happening again, or make a slide show if that's easier for you. Are you in the movie or observing yourself...any colors, any music? Can you put sound to it? It's ok if you don't choose to have sound. Can you once again experience the good feelings? OK, Good. Now say to yourself: **"Yeah, I can do this"** and say it like you mean it...NOW!

Now I want you to think of yourself as if you are already thin in your mind. Go ahead and put your favorite outfit on and notice it's not tight. Do this now. You can think about it for the next 10 years, but unless you **do it** .... it won't make a difference **now**, will it? Feel all the excitement and be proud of how thin you are in your mind. How thin are you in your ultimate desire? You cannot fail when you do this every day...and why not? OK, are you there at your thinnest? Check it out, what do you see on the screen? Now say to yourself "YEAH", I can do this, so that you can feel it to the bottom of your stomach, the same way you felt your success before.

Take 3 deep breaths now, and let the air out slowly. Do it, do it, do it NOW! When you are having a learning experience that is interesting to you now say "AHA" because you can know you are one step further to becoming your **desired** size and weight. How do you know this possible? Because you have just grown in knowledge how to do it and you made the experience yourself. Do it again and again. "Repetition is the mother of invention". Practice makes perfect...well, almost.

Now I ask you: "During this experiment were you feeling A: disgusted, powerless and depressed? Or B: motivated, playful and curious? Or A and B (all of the above)? GOOD! You are on the way. All of your feelings give the "Aha" response.

Desire towards an outcome comes from a thought, and gives movement towards unleashing a possibility. Desire and the **passion** that accompanies desire, opens a new door and literally gives thought a heart beat. Desire by itself stimulates a trust into a new realm of being that gives pleasure to the beholder and a thirst for knowledge to create momentum towards and outcome. A mild interest usually isn't enough to carry an idea forward, but desire like a thirst unquenched can carry a thought to completion and satisfaction of the result, or outcome.

Sequence of events from original thought to taking action and actually losing the weight.

| | | |
|---|---|---|
| First the | **Thought** | "I'd like to be thin" |
| Second the | **Idea** | of possibility of being thin |
| | **Imagination** | about idea and possibility |
| In imagination a | **Picture** | formed of being thin |
| In this picture | **Feeling** | I felt excited about seeing |
| myself | | thin |
| Feeling | **Desire** | created desire to make it |
| happen | | |
| Desire | **Focus** | set up repeated thoughts or |
| the | | focusing of attention |
| on becoming | | thin |
| Was the feeling so good | | |
| and desire so great | **Outcome** | was formed |
| | **Persistence** | forming outcome created |
| continuous | | a c t i o n |
| toward possibility | | |

| Once outcome | | | |
|---|---|---|---|
| was formed a | **Decision** | | was made to take action |
| Decision caused | **State** | | or attitude |
| More | **Focus** | | |
| on | **Desire** | | caused desired state of being |
| your | | | ideal weight |
| | | | |
| Desire created | **Feeling** | | |
| | **Visualization** | | |
| | **Imagination** | | set up state of continuous |
| action | | | toward being thin |
| | **Will** | | |

# Chapter 3

## Know your Outcome and then detach from it

As the story of Alice in Wonderland goes, Alice was walking on the path one sunny day and came to a fork in the road. She wondered to herself: "Which road should I take now"? Should I go to the right, or to the left? When high on a fence post she saw a large white and pink caterpillar, and to Alice this caterpillar seemed very old and wise, and so she asked him: "Wise old caterpillar, can you tell me which road I should take? I don't know which one is the best for me". The wise old caterpillar took off his sunglasses and thought for a moment and then he said to Alice in a very old and wise tone: "Alice, where are you going?" and Alice, astonished by his question, said: "Oh mister wise old caterpillar, I don't know". And Mr. wise old caterpillar said: "HMMMMM" and put his sunglasses back on. Then he thought again for a moment and said: "Alice, if you don't know where you are going, it doesn't matter which road you take".

This chapter is about what you want!
Number 1... know your outcome
Number 2... know your outcome
Number 3... know your outcome

I think this is the first and most important step you can and must take. Let's take this step very seriously, and enjoy taking it.

When you concentrate on your personal and specific outcome of losing weight, your mind creates and opens the door to the possibility and creates the direction of reaching your desired goal.

Think about and focus now on your outcome of losing weight as if you have already attained it. Give this some time, and have fun imagining your desired outcome.

Write this down for this will be the guideline to work from every day, if only in your imagination.

1. How much weight are you willing to lose? How much are you going to lose? There is a good reason to know exactly how much you want to lose as this thought creates the motivation you need to take action. You are giving a suggestion to your subconscious.

2. Determine exactly what you will do to lose this weight. What are you willing to give, and how much are you willing to focus on your goal.(We do not get something for nothing) In other words, there are no free lunches! You can lose weight, by knowing exactly what you want, and taking action, even if you don't believe it yet.

3. Establish when you will have lost your desired amount of weight. Give yourself flexibility to lose 6 or 8 or 10 pounds per month.

4. Create a plan and begin that plan NOW; putting it into action stimulates your physical body. It only works when **you do it !**
   Think about your outcome. Focus on it. If your desire is not there now, remember when you had so much desire to lose weight that you would give anything to make it come true. Stand in the mirror then ask yourself: "Do I really care if I am fat?" And be honest with yourself. You can be thin and you can not fail if you continue to take action as you plan. Your

motivation sets up the desire to take action and to do your plan that you have said you are **willing to do.**

In order to win at being thin, you must have your outcome...your purpose defined...and for you **losing is letting go.**

Now, you may know your outcome and still have doubts about this challenge in the beginning. There are long time old habits to break and you may suffer a loss...of old comfortable habits such as eating large amounts of food with second servings and lots of dessert. So let go of the outcome and continue to follow your desire today!

Some days you may think it's just not worth it especially if you should encounter a disappointment in the course of a day. The first thing you may want to do is reach for chocolate or potato chips...your favorite fullfiller...and you may even give in to an old pattern only to feel guilty and this feeling guilty could lead you to another piece of...what ever is nearest to your hand to reach out and grab and put in your mouth...to get fullfilled.

INSTEAD ....

take those desperate moments and the money you were going to spend buying a chocolate and call a friend and tell them you chose to call them because you are feeling like eating when you're not hungry and feeling out of control and you are ready to eat to satisfy your guilty, lonely, angry feelings and you called them to let them know how important they are to you and you need their friendship. Ask for support. Call me! Reach out!

Divert and dissociate from thinking about food to satisfy your needs and begin to think of your new purpose in life in other areas such as...

*Partnership and relationships.* What is your outcome in a relationship in the next year…in the next 10 years? How can you enhance the one you are ??

*Personal Development.* Who do you want to become in the next 5 years? What hobbies and challenges do you want to have fun experiencing?

*Career.* What is your outcome in the working world? In the next 5 years, 10, 20? Is there something you have always wanted to do? It's not too late to have many new beginnings.

Thinking about your other desires, possibilities and outcomes, **distracts** you from thinking about reaching for a juicy piece of something to eat. You can say it's **food for thought!** How successful are you going to become in each one of the above areas? Write it all down, while you are thinking about it…and you know what? You start to take action in those areas, too…at least in your imagination! And as you learn how to lose weight and follow this program you will be able to transfer your new learning into other areas as well to meet other new goals.

The impulse to go for chocolate or what ever food it is for you…will pass. The impulse will pass…the impulse will pass…say it…"this impulse will pass".

Fill your gap with thinking about all your successes, get high on yourself and eat a carrott or two or three, or an apple or two if you really need to eat, and the impulse will pass. **Do it** and you have won the power over an impulse. You didn't want to be powerless to a piece of chocolate, did you?

Who you become in the process of achieving your goal of being your desired self is the real purpose. The real you. The feeling of being in control, the feeling of learning how you think, how you respond to your environment and its influence and how to stay on track toward your goal and carry it to completion is your own private secret to success. It's wonderful to know that you have all the resources you need within yourself. And when you know yourself better and understand and accept how you got to be the way you are, you can clear out the past and go forward. Each day you come closer to your outcome, you have a success. If you slip backwards you take a moment or two to ask yourself what is happening here? What do I need?

Figure it out and be thankful you realized what causes backslides. Call a friend, go back to the beginning of this book and trust yourself that you will get a message, an insight (an "AHA") from you unconscious. Listen to a tape again, take a walk, breathe. Perhaps that's all it takes to get back on track.

Added tips to keep you moving toward your goal:

Live in the moment

Keep your plan simple

Focus on your desire to stay charged by thinking of your small successes or big successes

Exercise daily even if it's a 30 minute walk or swim

Enjoy the state of feeling consistent, of giving yourself what you need

Notice each day how it feels to be successful, very little successes count!

Ask yourself who is doing this and observe yourself doing your desire

Make a daily menu of possibilities. Each day set aside a time and ask yourself...How do I know I'm successful today? Clue it is always about a feeling.

Notice how easy it is to feel good about your success. Real success is losing weight and gaining pleasure every day.

Remember all the good things that are happening today.

If you're not going in the direction you want, change the direction!

You are the choice maker!

Give yourself shiny eyes and butterflies in your stomach every day.

Every mental action creates a physical action, every physical action creates an affect, every affect creates a direction and direction takes you toward being your ideal weight forever. It's the heart muscle your developing, to give yourself **your hearts desire.**

A friend once asked Mike Tyson: "Mike how have you developed those muscles?" and Mike said: "I just push against the resistance. I stretch myself further than I think I can go every day, and when I feel like stopping I give in to resistance.

Push against your own resistance today. You can do it!

You are responsible for your world. If you are feeling blue that means events are controlling you. Sit quiet for some minutes and ask your heart: "What do I really want?". Then wait. An answer will come very quickly.

Delays are only excuses and procrastination is nothing but a ritual. It takes a lot of wasted energy to wait until next monday! Why not concentrate on taking action to reach your goal instead? Ask yourself: "If I don't do this, what will be the ultimate price?" and "If I do this now how much better would I feel?".

Be honest with yourself.

Procrastination causes you to avoid pain and if you want this weight loss to be permanent, you can realize that it is more painful to stay fat than it is to change, and taking that one step further, your desired change to be your ideal weight is a pleasure.

How would you be if you were being the best that you are?

Why do goals or outcomes work?

1.   Because as you think, so you become. If you focus on something, you'll experience it even at first in your imagination.
2.   Making a goal is to tell the unconscious and conscious minds where you want to be.

Write down all you will gain by reaching your outcome.

Write down what it will cost to not reach it.

Follow these steps for a well formed outcome and write all of this down. While you are writing list every **good feeling** you are having in the process.

1.   What do you want specifically?
2:   What is the outcome of getting this outcome? How will it affect your life?
3.   What would demonstrate you have gotten your outcome?
4.   What will you see when you are thin? (Anything that comes to your mind is fine). What, where and with whom do you want to experience your desired outcome? How will it effect your life? What will happen if you get what you want? List all emotions? How do you know the outcome is worth getting? It's a feeling of well being, right?

Now as you focus on your goal of losing weight, write down one action you can take today. What action can you take in this next week? What action are you going to take that you haven't taken in the past? Are you willing to follow this plan? What are you willing to give to reach your goal?

Set a time each day to re read this chapter. This is an outline, a first step, a beginning of change for you!

I encourage you to **follow** now, and soon you will be **leading** yourself to success.

Since this guideline is very important take all the time you need to carry on a communication with yourself about answering each question precisely and accurately.

The importance for this is so that you will know each day that you are successful as you take responsibility for following your plan!

Some of the answers will surprise and delight you, so have fun with yourself as you write your guideline. Then follow along each day watching it happen.

# Chapter 4

## Imagination creates our power and our state of possibility

The aspect of human beings that sets us off from all other creatures is that of imaginative wisdom. Animals see things as they are, but we see them as they can be. We have been given the ability to transform. I have never seen anything give a person as much energy as a vision that he or she is developing to bring into reality. I have seen people forsake sleep, food and comfort for the sake of a project that they love. I can remember for myself also, once I had a vision of being my ideal self and realized the possibility, I was unstoppable. There is something very magic about a person dedicated to a purpose, something more precious than I can attempt to put into words. It is the miracle of creation. It is exactly this miracle which enables us to transcend circumstances. The same energy that moved the Einsteins and the Edisons **to change the world is within us.** We have an inspiration, a thought, inside ourselves that draws us to our own excellence if we are willing to listen and act on it. Within you lie talents far greater than you have recognized and expressed, and it is your imagination that causes you to trigger a possibility. What I mean by that is, whatever you can imagine is possible for you to create and when you imagine yourself as you desire, as if it has already become a reality, you are giving a signal to the unconscious that you are ready to be what and who you want to be.

And when you see yourself in your imagination this not only causes you to think about your possibilities but you realize you are capable of becoming your desired self. It is the simple law of cause and effect. Imagination is literally the workshop of the mind. If you think about it, all plans of losing weight have been fashioned in your mind. Your limitation for losing weight in the past is *in the past* and lies in the use of your memory. It no longer exists.

Here's how I think it works: through creative imagination your mind has direct contact with your unconscious. It is the faculty through which hunches and inspirations are received and it is through creative imagination that all basic or new ideas come to you. The creative imagination functions only when the conscious mind is working as a chain reaction, such as when the conscious mind is stimulated through the emotion of a strong desire. Also that creative imagination becomes more alert through use. Just as any muscle or organ of the body develops through use. Your imagination is first only a thought and of no value until it has been transformed into its physical counterpart. So while you are actively working on this program to lose weight, should you slip backwards into old habits, you can get right back on track by going back to your imagined self to create the desire that puts your cause back in motion. You are the driver of your own bus, so to speak.

Transformation of your imagination and desire creates your physical body to move into the state of taking action. It really helps to write down your imaginative thoughts. You can have so much fun with your own imagination, as you imagine yourself in the kind of clothes you will be wearing. You can even plan a new way you want to look, which colors you will be wearing, and how will you feel when people begin to notice the change in you. You can imagine what you will say to them, and how you want to stand, and it is through your imagining yourself in your new clothes that you set up once again your physical body to take action. It triggers possibility. The thought of your own possibility creates the butterflies, the sparkling eyes.

I remember at the time I was deciding to lose weight that Calvin Klein Jeans were the thing to be wearing to be the most fashionable, and of course before that time I had never imagined I would ever be able to wear a pair, because I was too fat. However when I saw myself in my imagination in jeans size 10, I had so much desire to reach my goal that one day I bought a pair of Calvin Klein Jeans in a size 10 and proceeded to grow into them. I'll never forget the day I actually got them up over my hips with about 4 inches of my fat stomach standing in the way of closing the zipper. And then one day I thought: "I'll just see how I've graduated to zipping those jeans up", and much to my astonishmet I closed them and even buttoned them at the top. I couldn't sit down though yet, so I took them off, hung them on the closet door and looked at them every day for 3 more weeks. And then one day it happened. In those days I had heard that it was very in Vogue to wear them so tight that some women even had to lay down on the bed to zip up their jeans, so I thought if necessary I would follow suit. I smile to myself now when I think how much desire I had to get into those jeans! To my surprise I didn't even have to lay down. As I closed the zipper *and* the button, I looked at myself in the mirror and gave a yell! "Yeah". Instant goose bumps! The feeling of reaching my goal and the pleasure of how I looked to myself was to great to ever go back to anything less. And as I made a commitment to me I have never gone back to old habits of eating and eating and eating, where I would not take responsibility for feeling good about me. My positive state further encouraged me to notice that I was in charge. I began to wonder why I had weighted (waited so long), and I realized it was because up until then I hadn't believed in myself and my capabilities. The particular state I came to know was one of **confidence, inner strength** and **ecstasy**, and these enabling states tapped the iceberg of my personal power. Later I learned that our behavior is the result of the state we are actually in. The key then is to **take charge** of our imagination, of our **states** and of our behavior that follows. And the key to our power is **taking action!** Taking action! Taking action!

Let me give you an example of just what a state is. It is our response to a happening or an event in our daily lives. If we receive a telephone call that we have just won the lottery, your response is one of excitement and elation. If you want confidence or excitement, they are states that you create in your imagination. You produce these states within yourself. Take love for example. If we want love in our life, it is first a thought and then a feeling about how fulfilling it would be to be in love. Your imagination is an attempt to satisfy your needs in advance, and therefore take action toward getting your needs met.

You have learned now about the components of imagination, and you see that you are capable of imagining yourself how you want to be. However, if you only think and imagine your outcome, you can think and think, and nothing happens. Action comes from a feeling of delight even if only in your imagination. You just are propelled into taking action!

When you have made your mind clear about how much weight you will lose and how long you want it to take, the most important of all is that *you make the decision* to get what you want. You will find yourself asking, why didn't I make that decision a long time ago? It was waiting for you all the time. Once you make this decision you can already see yourself. So an idea is an impulse of thought that impels action by an appeal to the imagination and ultimately a feeling in your heart of delight about your own possibility.

In the previous chapter you found out what you really want for you. You now know the amount of weight you desire to lose, when you want to accomplish your goal, and you have asked yourself the question: "What am I willing to give to get what I want?". Now I ask you to reverse your thinking and ask yourself the question: "What do I not want?". When you think about how much you don't want to be overweight, what happens? Perhaps you begin to feel angry that you are fat, or angry at others for contributing (however well meaning) to your dilema of not feeling as you would like to, or perhaps you begin to think how uncomfortable you can bee about trying and trying to lose weight to no avail, or having lost weight before and then gaining it back. If you look at yourself honestly in the mirror, you can feel and see the condition of uneasiness and here I want to say it is so important to go ahead and feel all the feelings even if they are uncomfortable, because a state or a condition of confusion or discomfort can be very useful, although uncomfortable for a while. When this feeling gathers more strength, it can be just the trigger that causes you to move onto the next necessary state of mind which is making an **absolute decision,** a decision that you absolutely will not tolerate or accept an overweight condition. If this is true for you it is now important for you to make a big decision. Here you can say to yourself something like this: "I no longer accept or tolerate being fat". Say it to yourself as you stand in the mirror. And shout it to the top of your lungs if necessary until you are clear with yourself. If you say "I'll try, or next month, or next January, or one day..... maybe...it won't work, unless you convince yourself. If you knew you could not fail, would you make that decision now?

To make this decision is to direct your thoughts and desires directly into action. Many of the problems in our lives are not a result of wrong choices, but of lack of making a choice. The stakes in the way we make decisions are high. If we decide with surety, clarity and resolution, we get what we decide for. If we flounder in indecision and procrastination, we lose our power. If we really want to create movement in our lives, we must be willing to take a sure step in one direction. We know all we need to know to make any decision for ourselves...and you make your decision to lose weight. If you make an error then admit it, learn from it and go on.

How do we make decisions? The decisions we make in our lives, lead us down the road to pain or pleasure as the result following our decision.

So you ask yourself: "What does it mean to me to be thin?" and then you follow by asking the question: "What does it mean to me to be overweight?".

When you have that answer, you become clear with yourself. What we know about pain and pleasure is, we will do almost anything to avoid pain and anything that we know of to gain pleasure in all areas of our lives.

The decision point comes when what we are doing or attempting to do causes more pain than changing. When we can realize that change causes us to move in a direction that creates pleasure and well being, then we can't not do that which will give us relief or we stay stuck in pain. It is a process of finding out what we need to avoid, eliminate or reduce pain... or to create, amplify or secure pleasure. This process enables our freedom.

We feel pain through what we associate that was painful in the past. For instance, in mending or repairing a relationship, if you think about all the painful discussions and how one caused pain to another, it makes it more difficult to reunite. When you are now making your decision to lose weight, if you think of all the pain connected to being fat, your energy system to go forward can shut down, and you become anchored to past pain. In other words, your brain links pain or pleasure to an event and a feeling. These negative and positive associations can cause you to change your direction. For example anger associated to an event can cause you to not face the issue and to avoid solving the problem, because of the fear of experiencing the pain. In reality it is action that changes our direction toward pleasure, not events. And before all action comes a decision. Decision gives direction. That is, it is the determining factor in what to focus on. When we focus on past pain, that's what we get, pain. When you focus on becoming slim, you have made the decision to not go back to past pain, because you begin to realize that being the new you means pleasure. The decision turns your thinking around to a curiosity of what you can do to become how you want to be and have pleasure.

Are you ready to make the decision? This means to rule out all possibility to be fat. You say to yourself, I absolutely give up being overweight, I will no longer interfere with my pleasure of well being.

Remember 5 good decisions you made in the past and how those decisions affected your life.

Now think about 5 decisions you didn't make that caused you pain.

Next think of 5 decisions you made that led you to making more and more decisions until you felt good. Take time for this, as it is an important step in your losing weight process.

Not making a decision is also making the choice to not take action. Not making a decision can also mean you have a fear, be it fear of failure or fear of success.

You always know all you need to know to make any decision with which you are confronted. Time spent in regretting a decision you didn't make before is only more time wasted. That's all.

Onother helpful hint for overcoming making a decision is to listen to your inner voice. You need to be quiet to hear what is inside yourself. Worry or fear creates mental and emotional states that block our awareness.

When I decided to give up being fat, I was already 40 years old. A friend said to me one day on the way to the beach (as I was bemoaning how I looked in my bathing suit): "When are you going to give up being fat?" I said: "What do you mean?. It's not that easy". Later I thought, it really was that easy, for when I made the decision to ask for help…to take action, it was the beginning.

Every decision takes courage, because we face the unknown and we put off these decisions because we fear we will fail. But the truth is that when you make your decision. You take charge of your life. You are already being courageous enough to direct your life for you. You deserve the best of all that you already are.

# Chapter 5

# *Life happens As You Believe*

In the bible it says: "Life Happens as You Believe" and so if you have the faith of mustard seed you can move mountains. As a child I wondered what all that meant, and I even wore a mustard seed around my neck, just in case it worked even if I didn't understand. Faith in what? It doesn't say exactly, but over the years I began to try to untangle this beautiful metaphor that people all over the world for thousands of years have lived their lives, or at least tried to, and I wondered "What about faith in yourself?". If you believed in yourself, could you remove obstacles in your life? Let's find out. Hmmm…If I believe I can be a person with 130 pounds, could that belief help me?

You've heard the saying *I'll believe it when I see it*, which means every thought must be proven in order to be real. Dr Wayne Dyer titled his book *I'll see it when I believe it*. That title stuck in my brain and it meant to me that we must *first believe* in order for results to be possible. Tony Robbins says: "A belief is nothing but a state, an internal representation that governs behavior". It can be a belief in possibility, a belief we will succeed or achieve something or it can be a belief that we can't succeed. If you believe in success, you will be empowered to achieve it. If you believe in failure, those messages will lead you to that experience as well. You have choices and *you can choose beliefs that limit you* or you can *choose beliefs that support you.* Where do beliefs come from, and why do some people have beliefs that push them toward success, and others have beliefs that help them to fail? For example: I can't do this today! Notice all the feelings that come as a result of this belief. Now try this: I can do this today! Say it! Now notice the new feelings. Just notice and observe. These two statements certainly create two complete different feelings. One of possibility and the other of dispair.

As you continue finding out information in this book about setting up the conditions for taking action toward your desired outcome, you may be thinking positively or negatively about your own possibilities and capabilities. At one time perhaps a thought will come into your mind "I can do this weight loss program" or "I can't do this weight loss program" for various reasons. By definition, *a belief is a feeling of certainty about an idea you feel is true.*

If you say: "I can do that" your belief in possibility delivers a direct command to your nervous system and when you believe you can really lose weight you go into the state of its being true. If you say you can or if you say you can't..... you are right. Your belief directs your reality.

Let's find out if you have any limiting beliefs about your being able to lose weight. Ask yourself the following questions and write down your answers in this book.

Here are the questions. Write them down.

What do you really want? ...

How do you want to achieve your heart's desire? ....

What do you want to experience when you have reached your weight at ...? ...

Ask yourself these questions 5 times and write down the first answer that comes to your mind, even if the answer changes somewhat.

Now...in order to find out any limiting beliefs, you ask yourself this question:

Why haven't I lost weight in the past?

Take some very important moments for yourself to *honestly* answer.

What happened when I tried to lose the weight before?

Here are some examples of limiting beliefs I have heard from others. These will help you find your own limiting beliefs.

I can't lose weight because I'm just like my mother and she is fat.

I can't lose weight because I must cook for the children and eat with them to form a good example.

I can't lose weight because I must entertain many people at dinner parties.

I can't lose weight because I have a big bone structure.

I can't lose weight because all the people in my family are big.

I can't lose weight because I'm lazy.

I can't lose weight because I just look at sweets and gain weight.

I can't exercise because I don't have time.

Everytime I lose weight I gain it back.

Now write down your own.

Now what beliefs do you need to make your ideal weight a reality?

Here are some examples:

I can lose weight and reach my goal because I am committed to myself

I can lose weight by following my plan. Small steps count.

I can lose weight by taking responsibility for my decision each day. A new decision a new beginning

I believe means I can do it

I believe I am capable

I believe I can create my own reality

I can do this. (This is the most powerful belief of all)

Try it on for size.

Where do beliefs come from?
Beliefs come from messages we received from our parents and others in the environment where we grew up. Some beliefs we learned as children:
"Only the rich get richer, and the poor get poorer"
"Food must never be thrown away"
"We must clean our plates"
"Children must obey their parents or be punished"
"Girls are not as strong as boys" (Really an old belief, Ha!)

With every limiting belief there is a positive intention. This positive intention was mostly to please our parents, because in the primary years, we can only know ourselves in the mirroring eyes of our caretakers. The only way a child has of developing a sense of self is through a relationship with another. We are *we* before we are *I*. The other persons, our primary caretakers become significant in the sense that person's love, respect and care for us really matter. As a child grows older, he or she, begins the process of forming their own identity, and they are in a process of "holding on and letting go". The old beliefs about eating habits may continue even when a person realizes they are stuck in their old ways, because reigning supreme is for every person to get those primary needs met, and to please their parents. Often eating for fulfillment answers these needs, because eating behaviors were rewarded in the past.

My mother is a great cookie maker and cake maker. In fact, many times I 've seen my mother busily making cookies to carry down the street to someone who was ill or sad and lonely. She baked cookies for church functions, social gatherings and school functions, in fact I can never remember a time when there wasn't a cookie in the house for they were always stored in cookie tins of various sizes and shapes, to be offered if someone should drop in for coffee. For years and years conversations were centered around the kitchen table with coffee and plates of cookies. Needless to say I also consumed hundreds or maybe thousands of cookies over the years while solving problems or emotional issues with absolutely no notion that these delights were contributing to my ever growing problem of weight control. I too, began baking cookies, and believed they were contributing to soothing pain or hurtful feelings. These beliefs turn into habits that can give comfort for a life time without even realizing the side effects. Believe me, I'm not saying we should rule out cookies from our lives, by any means my point here is to begin to realize and interpret how we use food which can contribute to beliefs that we can't lose weight. If you believed it was neccessary to eat while solving problems then that belief can be associated to thinking you can solve problems by eating, or that with eating the problems will temporarily go away.

Since it has become important for you to lose weight now, it is necessary to become aware of old beliefs around your eating, and substitute them with new supportive beliefs. So what would you need to believe about yourself in order to assure yourself that you cannot fail?

Try these. Select one or more that you can say to yourself with conviction.

I believe I can lose weight

I am gaining freedom from old habits

I am my own best friend

Every thought I have is a cause set in motion.

No one is lazy, they are just uninspired or have lost interest.

I am responsible for my decision to lose weight

I can do this step by step. Small steps count!

Here is an example of installing a positive belief system with a weightloss client.

Mary:     Now that you have made the decision to lose weight, Hans, how are you going to proceed so that you are absolutely certain you cannot fail?

Hans:     I believe in Arnold Schwartznegger. He is who I look up to and my role model for losing weight. He says: "You do it step by step. (Belief) The more you do it the more fun you have. (Belief)".

(Here Hans substitutes the beliefs of others who are successful. Lee Iococa is also a role model for Hans)

Mary:     What does Lee do? What is his secret?

Hans:     Lee says: "When your down and you don't think you're going to make it, keep on going and it will get lighter and lighter".

Mary:     Hans, how do you do this every day?

Hans:     I only think of my desired weight.

Mary:     What do you think about when you have the body you want?

Hans:     I think about what I can lose and what I can win. (Belief)

Mary:     What more can you do?

Hans:     If I fall off track, I look to others and see how they maintain healthy bodies. I picture their bodies and study how they do it.

Mary:     How old is the person in your picture?

Hans:     42 years old, the same as me.

Mary:     What would happen if you didn't keep on going?

Hans:     I think about all the pain I will continue to have.

Mary:     What will you be doing tomorrow?

Hans:     I will be losing weight step by step. (Belief)
    I will picture others. (Role modelling Chap. 9)

| Mary: | When you use these beliefs can you stay on track? |
| --- | --- |
| Hans: | Yes, I can do that. (Belief) |
| Mary: | So Hans, here are also some helpful resources. I am going ask you to take action now that you believe you can. Put a picture on your bureau of someone, like Arnold, and below it write down the steps you can do every day. If you find yourself in doubt or fear about your success with weight loss you have a picture of yourself overweight under the other picture. You can say to yourself, I used to believe...and substitute your old limiting belief .... but now I believe...My example: If others can successfully lose weight, I can too. And here is my favorite new belief: I am a visionary in action, and I am transcending my history of being overweight. |

By the way, Hans now believes in himself, and has directed his state to that of becoming 40 pounds less.

After Hans lost 40 pounds I asked him: "Hans, what is most important about your having done that?". He said: "I found out I needed help and support from others". Mary: "What else?"

| Hans: | "I found out I had to have love from others, so that I would feel important even when I am smaller. I had learned when I was a child, big people have a better chance in life (Belief)". |
| --- | --- |

And now ask yourself if you BELIEVE the following questions?

1. Do you believe everything you think or do is a cause set in motion?
2. Do you believe every thought and action is going to have an effect on you?...and a result?
3. Do you believe results stack up to take your life in a particular direction?
4. Do you believe for every direction there is a destination?

Now let's see what happens when you hold on to your old limiting beliefs.

Imagine it is 1 year from now and you are still overweight…and as if it were already one year from now. Notice where you are and who you are with, what you are wearing and what you are telling yourself, like: "I just can't seem to lose weight, and already it's one year later" and in your imagination notice how that feels to be still uncomfortable.

And now imagine it's 2 years from now. Picture that now. Who is there with you, and how does that feel when you still believe it's not possible to lose weight and be happy with yourself? Now imagine it's 3 years from now, and you still haven't lost weight. In your imagination have you given up?

Now in this exercise let's substitute your new beliefs. Notice the difference, and how your new beliefs motivate you to take action …

It's 1 year from now and you are really enjoying yourself because you have reached your desired weight. Where are you then, now in your imagination? And imagine you say to yourself: "I am my own best friend". And someone says to you: "How did you lose all that weight?" and you answer: "I am a visionary in action and I'm just living my dream.". Notice how that feels in your imagination as if it were already true.

And now it's 2 years from now and you are enjoying yourself in your freedom from old habits of being fat. And a person says to you: "You look great.What is your secret?". And you answer: "With a new belief such as I am responsible for my weight loss and I choose to feel good about me". Notice how you feel.

Now it's 3 years in the future and you have even reached more goals in other areas as a result of your knowledge for losing weight. Someone says to you: "What happened to you when you lost all that weight?…You seem like a different person.". And you say: "I learned I can believe in myself because I have everything I need to reach my goals inside myself". Just take a moment or two to acknowledge how that feels in the future now, as you picture yourself 3 years from now as if it is already true, saying to yourself "YES".

Our imagination can be so delightful! Right?

# Chapter 6

## Fear

Fear is an illusion of possibility of an event occuring that relates to the past. And fear is about an imagined event in the future that hasn't even happened yet. I truly believe fear is about loss or imagined loss. If we have total success, the fear becomes one of losing what we have gained…and in weight loss, of gaining back what you have lost, which means losing the fight with yourself. Fear of either success with your weight loss program, or failure to reach your goal can be paralyzing and block your motivation to reach your goal, and it is based on what we believe to be true about ourselves based on past experiences. In other words, if we fear our success or fear our failure it only means we haven't suceeded in the past. So we are fearful of the future because of our past. But we are not now in the past. So what we are fearing is only *a memory of past experiences*. Since we have choices, we can experience new learning, experience our new ways of being and therefore the new results! Small steps count!

For some people, living their dream must include giving up something or sacrificing as they are striving to reach their goal, even after they have reached it! I heard a participant in one of my courses saying to me: "I'm afraid that when I reach my desired weight I will leave my husband. I have only stayed with him because I thought no one else would want me!"

Or: "I'm afraid when I have lost my weight, I will have the opportunity to be in a relationship, and I'm afraid to become close to anyone".

Or: "I'm afraid if I become small I will not receive love .... I was an accident!" Later he overheard a conversation when he was a little boy between members of his family who spoke fondly about him only as they were saying he was just like Grandfather who died 2 weeks before he was born. It seems that grandfather was a big fat and jolly type man and wanted to live to see this young child be born. The whole family loved this big fat grandpa and my client was an unwanted child. Somehow either unconsciously or consciously he connected that if he were like this grandfather he also would receive love even though he was unwanted. Big was what he associated with (fat and jolly), and all his life he ate all he could to receive love. Later when he was attempting to lose weight, he wanted to find a loving relationship and felt this was not possible weighing 320 pounds. He began to lose weight and during the process he found a girlfriend. His weight loss ceased temporarily because he once again realized he was eating for love, and with a girlfriend who loved him...being fat didn't matter...in fact he felt powerful and protecting toward her just like...grandpa. It was only when he feared losing her that he got confused and came to therapy.

He realized that the fear of losing this love was causing him to eat compulsively again because of how he related to the past.

This very fear can cause one to self defeat because it would leave them open to deeper **fears of loss**. Fear can be a warning signal to us, or a friend protecting us from being unsafe. Either way, we need to become aware of our fears, and learn how to channel them into a direction where we are safe and open to understanding the real issues underneath. Fear is nothing but a temporary state of mind, and you have already learned that you can redirect **yourself** from one state of being to another through your imagination.

So if you can direct your thoughts…and your state of mind…and its equivalent state of physical being, you can also redirect your fears. Remember the driving force is your desire. It is time now that I challenge you to stay true to your desire while overcoming your fears.

Loss causes pain, and the fear of loss causes us pain in advance of the imagined loss. Loss can cause pain no matter if we lose our dog, a loved one or our youth. Many persons have in the past lost their parent's love through abandonment or through shame (shame to be discussed in the next chapter). Often in families where little love is given, there is chronic distress, and every person in the family adapts to that stress in order to get their needs met. Each member becomes anxious and fearful. In such an environment it is difficult for anyone to get his basic human needs met. The major consequence of this chronic stress can be abandonment. What that means is there is no one there for the child, no mirroring to affirm that the child is good, and no one the child can depend on. The parents are often in their own conflict but the child doesn't know that and interprets either that they are unwanted or that something is their fault, because after all, they may have been an accident in the first place. When an excess of alcohol is evident in a family, or when mother and father are in conflict, it's virtually impossible for love to be given, or to even model self love. A child's needs for love and attention can not be met in this situation, so the child turns inward and ultimately to self indulging habits, and sometimes pain killers…which, as some of you know, can be **food**…since it brings temporary comfort.

When the family system is unbalanced, the children attempt to create a balance. The accidental child can feel emotional abandonment in the womb. Literally, the message is "we can't handle another child". What this really means is that children need their parent's time, attention, love and direction for at least 25 years. When they do not get these comforts, they can feel emotionally abandoned. According to John Bradshaw, in his studies on the family, abandonment sets up compulsivity. Since the children need their parents all the time, and since they do not get their needs met, they grow up with a "cup that has a hole in it". It is this hole in the soul that drives the person into being compulsive so as this person looks for more love, attention, and praise, he attempts to find false substitutes or other ways to mood alter. The drive comes from **emptiness.** I believe all compulsive behaviors are ways to **avoid** the pain of unacceptable feelings.

In order to avoid the **fear of loss** (losing one's parent through abandonment or loss of love) a child will deny or become delusional about what is happening in the family. He pretends and fantasizes everything is OK and he can recreate fulfilment with the feeling of eating (the altered state of conditions induced by emotional starving). In all compulsive behaviors, such as eating, the illusion of connection is restored, and one is not alone. Compulsive overeating is not about being hungry, it is about mood alteration. They distract us so we don't have to feel the lonliness and emptiness.

Here is an example of how compulsive eating begins. The Orange Family

Jack Orange, the father is authoritarian, rigid and controls his emotions. He also attempts to control the emotions of all those around him. Jack is an overachiever. He is a work addict and exactly like his father. Jack married Jonelli, who had a rigid and authoritarian mother. Jonelli has a weight problem. Through the years she has struggled with a fat, thin obsessive eating disorder. She stays so preoccupied with fat thinking that she can avoid her low grade depression, which is really anger directed inward. She is angry at herself for never standing up to her mother, and for staying in a marriage she wanted to leave long ago. She is also addicted to her husband in that she constantly thinks about how awful he is. She has no time to be in touch with her own feelings. She is really enraged at her husband and the mother's rage is equated with food. Mom has reenacted her own childhood by marrying someone controlling like her mother. Of course no one talks about their feelings, how they have low self worth, anger and lonliness. The only time the family even attempts to communicate is around the eating table, and in this family 2 children are overweight, one is anorexic.

Food in this family is the vehicle for feeling fulfilled, along with being the substitute for feeling their feelings.

The point here is that everyone stays in this situation because of fear of loss. They imagine that if they talked about their feelings and got some help that they would lose the family.

The fear of this imagined loss keeps them stuck or blocked because what is feared is to be left alone.

This is the place where change can occur or it can be repeated in the next generations. The point comes where there is so much pain and fear that it is realized that any change will be less painful than the existing situation...and this is the point where health can be restored. This specialized knowledge can enable you to finally break out of these old eating habits that are just too painful to live with anymore, and the best part about your knowing how eating disorders get started is that you know you can take charge because these fears however large or small can be redirected by learning how to manage your state of mind and of body. With this knowledge you can set yourself free.

The truth is...You can't lose anything...it always transforms.

You make loss up in your head...because remember...fear is an illusion about something that hasn't even happened...and 92 % of all the fears and worries we conjure up in our mind...don't happen. But believe me, I know the pain of the fear is always real, whether the feared event happens or not.

The best way to deal with your fears is to utilize them. Ask yourself the question: "How can I use this information?".
Answer:
1.   Change your focus to your desired outcome
2.   Think about all your new positive beliefs, and think about them and think about them and think about them, until you are convinced.
3.   Think about how grateful you are for finally being able to understand why you haven't lost weight before
4.   Realize that all of our caretakers, parents, grandmothers and grandfathers did their best
5.   Remember it's easier to blame others than face your own fears.

A woman came to me and said: "I hate myself and I can't lose weight" and I said to her: "How does that make you feel?". She said: "I feel trapped inside my body, lonely and like I'm cheating myself. I am settling for less that I know I can be. My boyfriend is thinking about leaving me and I feel terrible".

I said to her: "What must you believe about yourself to be fat?". She said: "I hate myself and I believe I don't deserve to be beautiful and vital. I don't deserve the love of this man, and I'm afraid I will lose it".

I said: "What kind of a woman do you want to be?". She said: "Energetic, motivated, productive and a loving example".

I said: "Have you ever been all those things before?". She said: "I have always been dependent on others". I said: "What must you believe to settle for less?". She said: "That I'm not important. That I am self conscious, and that I don't love myself and also that I must focus on others instead of myself". So I asked her to imagine herself physically fit, a productive worker and energetic, loving and fun and what would she have to believe to keep this person. She said: "I would have to be serious about my life, I would have to love myself and set an example. And to believe I deserve the best. I asked her what she was willing to do to have that person. She said learn to love herself every day.

When you don't live up to your standards you violate yourself.

I asked her what she was willing to do to lose weight and stop the fear of losing her relationship.

She said:

1.   I am willing to get up loving myself.
2.   I am willing to exercise
3.   I am willing to take myself seriously

I asked her:…"Can you do this?". She said: "**I can do this**".

As she took responsibility for herself I noticed she stopped saying *that person* about herself, and began to say *I*. Then I said: "Is that who you really are?". She said: "YES".

She had learned pain because of her fears, when the truth is she was blocked by fear. When she realized she already had everything she needed inside herself to have what she desired, she set herself free. Aren't we always looking for that which is already inside ourselves?

# Chapter 7

## *Shame*

If a child lives with criticism, he learns to criticize others. If a child lives with hostility, he learns to fight. If a child lives with shame, he learns to *feel ashamed*.

Too much shaming creates an internalized shame that is covered by obsessive control and perfectionism. All forms of psychological abuse are shaming, yelling, name calling, labeling, criticizing, judging, ridiculing, humiliating and comparing are all sources of shame. The most destructive aspect of shame is the process whereby shame moves from a feeling to a state of being or it is internalized. For example, when one is taught that anger is a sin, one becomes ashamed when he is angry. Calling children "bad", spanking and punishing them for being bad causes them shame. Shamed persons feel flawed and defective as human beings, and they can resort to mood altering substances or food to cover feelings of being "bad". And so, it is no surprise that an adult carrying out daily activities at home or in the work place, when criticized or put down for some activity will relate to being criticized in the past. And if food is his chosen instant gratifier the possibility is that he or she will run for the nearest quick fix which could be chocolate or sweets...for me potato chips, to dull the emotional pain.

It is important for you to be aware of these shaming consequences, because when you are aware and alert to these associations and patterns, it is much easier for you to realize what is happening…smile to yourself and say "AHA …this is the same old feeling of being not good enough"… and do something else that is not contributing to your being overweight. You can take action immediately by focusing on your goal, feeling the good feelings of already being thin which can change your emotional state…ask yourself the question "What am I feeling?".

And…don't forget to feel all the good feelings for your success in that moment.

Give yourself a mental hug and a lot of love. You deserve it.

I speak about shame in connection with weight loss because it is relevant to food addiction, in that one can form a bond with food that is otherwise missing in a relationship. There is a belief connected with this type of behavior of bonding with food, and that is that one is undesirable, and that no one could want or love them as they are. In fact they cannot love themselves. And it can follow that when love is not available, they might as well eat and eat and eat because it becomes the second best thing in giving comfort. Other beliefs can follow such as "I'll be OK if I eat". In other words "I need something outside to be whole". Now this shame way of thinking can begin as a child is being told they are making mistakes especially when  mistakes are not accepted in the family. They begin to think: "I am not accepted" or "I am a mistake" or "I am not acceptable as I am". A young person internalizes this blame and shame by thinking they are bad if they make a mistake, and furthermore, when they make a mistake and are bad they can no longer accept themselves. Included here, one can develop a disgust for one's body because a person associates unacceptance with being flawed. Worth is measured on the outside, and not on the inside.

The mental obsession about a specific addicitive relationship with food is first mood altering, since eating takes us out of our emotions. One may even eat secretly in a hiding place, and use food as the only way to temporary comfort. At this point personal worth is at its lowest. According to John Bradshaw, there is a difference between healthy guilt and shame. A person with guilt might say "I feel bad because I did something that violated my standards or values ..." or "I feel sorry about the consequences of my behavior" and in doing so the person's values and self esteem are reaffirmed. The possibility of repair exists and learning and growing are promoted. Guilt is a feeling of regret and responsibility for one's actions while shame is a painful feeling about oneself as a person. In a shame and food addiction situation the person involved is actually having a love affair with food. I say this because not only does food fill a love gap, it causes one to temporarily forget about his or her inner pain. At this point, escape from oneself is necessary because to face oneself causes the excruciating pain of facing one's alleged worthlessness. The person keeps herself in a state of disease whereby the authentic self is kept hidden or unknown. Sometimes a wall of fat will keep a person protected from another person seeing who they really are. Or in another sense, extra weight of great proportions can give a person more substance. It can help to not feel so small inside.

There is a young boy I know who was raised by a single parent as a result of a divorce. His father relocated to the other side of the country and this boy suffered as a result of not having his father's love and daily support. This was an athletic boy, a football player, and when he became an adolescent, he was the star of the football team and socially accepted and respected. He realizes the value of carrying extra weight because it added to his strengh in playing the game, but in addition to that, he received attention and rewards about his size from the other fathers of the boys of the team. They would fondly tell him he was really strong and that his size really made a good player. He received the missing love from his father through the other fathers and it also filled his needs when his father was not there to watch him play football. When his father left, the boy felt shame about the divorce, and a sense of abandonment with his father. His own self worth became associated with his father's leaving. When he got rewarded for being big and strong, he began to take in more food and became fat. And even after he left the school, his association with food and being a strong person continued. The association, the bond with food, had been established, and it was important for him to find his own self worth, his value within himself, before he could lose weight as he wanted to.

# Chapter 8

## *Values*

All of what you are learning works together to create a result. It is like a delightful recipe and so far you have these necessary ingredients.

You know everything begins with a thought or an idea and you had a thought and an idea of how great it would be to be thin, right? And the more you thought about it the more interesting it became, in fact you put it into the wish category and felt a desire to be slim and healthy. The more you thought about it the more you defined it and this wish and desire became a possibility if only in your mind. You found out exactly what you want to weight and when you want that to happen, and the more you imagined your outcome as if it had already happened, the more you wanted it, right? You realized when you wanted to be thin bad enough that you finally made a decision to redirect your wishes and desires with the knowledge that your result will happen when you believe in it. Learning about fear and what has blocked you in the past helped you with a new awareness that you can change those old patterns from the past, recognize the feelings that accompany your new knowledge about yourself and go forward with your plan to actualize your ideal weight. You are on your way to a healthy soup rather than stewing in the past!

How much time do you spend thinking about what is important to you? Here is a list of values most people say is of utmost importance to them. What is really important for you?

| | |
|---|---|
| Love | Friendship |
| Ecstasy | Harmony |
| Communication | Free time for you |
| Respect | Relaxation |
| Fun | Prestige |
| Support | Security |
| Challenge | Honesty |
| Creativity | Freedom |
| Growth | Spiritual unity |
| Beauty | Attraction |
| Affiliation | |

Look over this list carefully and consider which of these are important to you and then take a moment to rank order them from 1 being the most important to 10.

These values represent the states we can move toward to be happy. They are states we want to experience or avoid. They are our needs.

Example: When these important needs are gratified you can be more comfortable while you are losing weight.

One of my participants said to me: "After asking myself what is important to me, I realized when I don't have the feeling of love from another person, I become empty inside, and so I EAT. Food becomes my substitute for LOVE. So I have learned to satisfy my loving relationship in order to flow through my day without overeating".

These values are important to you, they are what you need in order to be fulfilled. For example: if security is important to you and your boss tells you he must lay off 100 people and you may be one of them, you may become very stressed. You may run out and find another job moving away from the possibility and if you associate a feeling of security with eating a lot of food and being secure in your warm home...that's what you will do.

As you are thinking about your values now, please do not delete what you already have and what is already good...and please be able to ask for what you need.

Here is an example for you to consider. Say to a partner or friend:

"I need your love today"

or

"I need to know you respect me just the way I am, that it's OK just to be me"

or

"I need the freedom to make my own decisions today in my own way".

Note: If you do what you have always done before to get your needs met, you'll get what you've always gotten.

All the parts must work together or the machine will break down...and the stress will seek its weakest part or point. When you are not meeting your needs, so that your body functions well, you have the possibility of overeating. Internal conflicts or behavior do not support your needs...therefore we can discover what has to happen to get what is important to us. This is the power of values or knowing what is important to us. When we do not move toward our values, we do not become fulfilled.

Take some time now…all you need, to write down what values you must experience in order to lose weight.

I'll give my own example: today I need courage, patience and confirmation. How do I know? I asked myself "What do I need?". Just as our eyes are the windows to our inner self, so our emotions are directing us to our heart. Ask your heart: "What do I need?". The heart gives loving answers and sometimes just aknowledging our love for others and for ourselves gives us the energy we need. "All things are simply unfolding even now". This helps with patience. And then tell your stories to a good friend. They most always will give you confirmation and love.

As the example before, what would cause you to not lose weight? Not having love…or security…or respect?

Values are our most powerful motivating tool, because when you are satisfied and content, and meeting your needs with what is important for you to be happy, the result is…you are fulfilled.

And finally here is a values list of important things to be aware of:
Procrastination
Finding fault with others
Focusing on Fears
Focusing on negative
Judging others
Holding on to the past

There is a saying in English…*no pain no gain*…and what it literally means is pain will force us to take a new direction because we are more motivated to avoid pain than we are to go toward pleasure.

Our reality is based on whatever we are focusing on. Here's an example of avoiding the pain and going toward what we value, toward what gives us pleasure.

I had a client who was addicted on chocolate, and she was successful in changing her habit of binging on chocolate everytime she was criticized. I said to her: "How did you not eat chocolate?". She said: "I made a picture (**focus on the outcome that is important**). I want to look good and feel better at a party in three months, and I thought about how my not taking action is going to be painful if I eat all this chocolate, so I saw myself just the way I wanted to look as if it had already happened, I dressed myself up in the most spectacular outfit I could imagine…and focused on it until it felt so good, I simply lost interest in the chocolate. I had changed my state and pulled myself out of that chocolate binge".

Sometimes when we are going toward our values we apply an approach avoidance technique. That means, we begin to go toward what gives us pleasure, but on the way, we become *afraid* for one reason or another. People are judging you or taking advantage of you and something causes you to not follow through with your positive intentions. This is where *focus* really comes in hand. You can turn it around by going back to focusing on what is important to you, which will contribute to changing your thinking about what is really important…what someone else said, or your desired outcome? Go back to what you believe about yourself…such as "I am my own best friend". I have all I need inside myself to be successful now.

Notice that you have more pain if you eat all that chocoalte than if you don't…and LINK YOUR PLEASURE TO NOT EATING IT!

Enjoy your soup, you are adding all the right ingredients.

Now that you know what is important to you, you can learn how to break those old patterns.

So let's use the example again of the person who avoided a chocolate binge. She interrupted her pattern of eating chocolate after being criticized, and that felt good, and she did it with her imagination and focus on herself at the party in a  outf it. She felt the pleasure of her success and decided to further interrupt her pattern of eating when she got to the party. So…she pictured herself at the party once again and this time she decided to not eat while she was there. Before she had hung around the food like it was the most important part of the gathering, but now she realized, what was really important was the conversation she would be having with the other guests. She saw herself not standing around the food, but finding interesting people to speak to. It felt good to her in her imagination, in advance, and so she put it into her plan of interrupting previous patterns.

Then she said to herself: "I'm a visionary in action. I'm transcending my history of eating too much food that I don't even need and I'm making my own decisions about what to focus on. How did I get so lucky?".

If you are noticing any doubts now or fears about your own success you know what to do.

1. What are you thinking?

2. Now ask yourself: "What do I really want?"

3. Am I still interested in my desire to be thin? When the answer is yes, then ask yourself what is stopping you. Write down the very next answer about what you think can stop you and that will be a limiting belief you still have. Like: "I've tried losing weight before but I failed". Then remember, you didn't fail, because there is no such thing, you just gave up then. That's it. Now think about your decision and install a new belief such as: "I can't fail" and notice how it changes your attitude. Take a deep breath. Yeah, do it now…and focus on your image of yourself as if it were already true. Feel the good feelings in advance and decide once again to **TAKE ACTION** knowing you want the pleasure of being at your ideal weight, right? All these little baby steps counts!

# Chapter 9

## Positive and negative emotions and the subconscious

All of the experiences we have affect and influence our conscious mind as well as our unconscious mind, and all experiences are recorded through our senses.

What is important to note here, is that we can become aware of our unconscious patternings that have become firmly set, and we can change the effect upon us by changing our behavior. The unconscious can be influenced by positive input through deep relaxation in a calm quiet state, and learning can take place with clarity. In a relaxed state, the mind is not cluttered with a mixture of thoughts.

Also, during relaxation, a calm sense of being with **yourself** can allow a sensation of accomplishment. Relaxation can enable you to approach a situation with a greater feeling of confidence. Not every relaxation is aimed at adding positive input to the unconscious. Some are meant to create awareness of feelings. While relaxing you are directed to the discovery or awareness of your own unconscious resources in order to change a situation not desired such as being overweight. Once you are aware of how you came to a state which caused you to gain weight to a point of being overweight, you can change simply through your intention or self suggestion. Until this awareness is reached, the old patterns of eating continue, and can result in a conscious feeling of being out of control. For this reason, the relaxation instructional tapes that accompany this book are useful while you are relaxing. You are learning to form new patterns.

The possibilities of creativity of thinking in the conscious state connected with the subsonscious mind can be inspiring and affirmative. When you accept as a reality the existence of the conscious mind transferring your desire and positive direction of weight loss into the unconscious, you can have confidence and trust in your results, for you are learning and training with your integrated thinking and awareness. It is something you can learn that creates insight and causes you to be motivated to take action. We all want to learn how to get motivated to be the best we are, right? And we do not want to stand in our own way or be blocked. It has been well established that we can give new suggestions to our inconscious mind and bring a new awareness to consciousness. It's the same as planting a seed and watching it grow and multiply.

We can also plant our intensions firmly in our hearts. They will also grow in our minds, and in our behaviors. It is a matter of cause and effect. For example if you squeeze an orange, what kind of juice do you get? The same is true: if you plant loving thoughts you reap loving emotions.

As you look at your inner world, it will reflect what is going on outside yourself. Everything begins inside you. It's true for all of us. If the engine of your car is not working, you don't go out and polish the car! Right? Rather you check the inner workings, the source of what makes your automobile run. In this regard you also go to your own source which is in a sense your unconscious source. Our feelings are energy in motion, e-motion. For example think a thought, reap an emotion.

What determines our emotions?

What we focus on.

What determines what we think about?

Our values .... That which is important to us. We strive all the time to get our needs met which lead us to pleasure and a sense of being fullfilled. From knowing what is important to us we direct ourselves to making decisions that lead to our feeling good.

Why are decisions nescessary?

To decide **not** to focus on what takes our power away

What determines our emotions?

When we focus on **fear** (we get what we focus on)

How can we turn old patterns into seeking new solutions?

Hold your intension as if you have already achieved it

**Emotion is created by motion**

When we delete our small steps of success we focus on what hasn't worked in the past our emotions also become like heavy weights on our body. As you begin to lose weight just notice your own light heartedness. Those lighthearted feelings motivate you.

THE SECRET

"Ask and you shall receive...seek and you shall find". You have all heard those famous quotes from the bible, and with the use of asking ourselves questions, we can turn old patterns into new patterns that get the results we want, and have the energy to take action or **e-motion** (Energy filled motion).

When a condition or event happens in your life, the first question to ask yourself is: "What does this mean?". All of life's meaning, is the meaning you give it. The answer to the question "What does this mean?". Does this event or circumstance or condition you find yourself in cause you **pain** or **pleasure**? We all will do our best to get away from pain, and go toward pleasure. Why? Because it feels good...and **all of us want to feel good!** So if we intend and give attention to our possibility to get our desired result, we feel good. And if we focus on what we didn't do in the past we have a tendence to beat ourselves up. You are bundles of energy in motion. I am a bundle of energy in motion.

So, here we go with how to turn the old e-motions into new awareness, new possibilities. So let's take a moment of awareness, new awareness. Ask yourself these questions when you find yourself with the munchies...or when you find yourself eating to fill an empty feeling.

Here are the questions to ask yourself to change your mental state of being and therefore your attitude. Also, what you ask for, you will find...and you have all the potential you need inside yourself to reach your desired weight! Check your engine! Get out your pen and paper and write your answers.

1.  What am I most happy about today?
2.  What could I be happy about if I really thought about it?
3.  What is it about this situation that makes me happy and gives me a good feeling? What about this situation caused me to have a lightheartedness inside myself?
4.  What is it about this learning experience that gives me joy?
5.  What could I do today to turn my problems or mistakes into a learning experience?
6.  Who will I see today that will make a difference in my life?
7.  What am I really delighted about?
    If you can't think of something ask ...
8.  What if I were delighted? What could I be delighted about?
9.  What am I grateful for today?
10. What am I satisfied with?
11. Who loves me and who do I love?
12  What has to happen today for me to feel light energy in motion?

You can write your answers right here in this book, because tomorrow you can look at your answers, ask the same questions again, and see if you come up with some different answers, and the next day, and the next day. And what if this became a habit, to begin each day and watch the blahs go away, beginning now. Get a tablet or a journal and keep track. Have fun with it. Look at it later and smile at yourself that it's working…go ahead and smile ahead of time…like now! And the biggest question of all, **why not???**

A woman came into me for counseling one time and the first question she asked me was: "Do you ever get depressed?". I said: "Sure!". She said to me: "Oh how depressing". I truly believe what we focus on, we become…and the labels we give ourselves give us either a good feeling or a feeling of non acceptance of who we are, which leads to what we become.

Here are some examples of focusing on the old outdated emotions: "I'm having a mid life crisis", "I have no confidence", "I'm so lonely", "Life is hard. It seems like I'm just running around getting nowhere". When you say that, watch what happens.

Now, make up questions to follow the above statements such as: "What does this mean when I say I'm lonely? What do I need? What can I learn about being lonely?". For example: I can learn to develop a more interesting social life. I can call someone. I can change this . I can take another path today. I can sit and do nothing, at least for a while.

Heres some more: "I'm so frustrated", "I'm confused and I just don't understand", "I'm disappointed".

These emotional statements are **giving up** statements. There have been several books written about our emotional states and the power they have over us. In the "emotional hostage", frustration, confusion and disappointment are absolutely necessary and useful. They are known as the "Pot Boilers". In other words these emotions are the learning and changing stimulators.

Are we afraid of our emotions? Do we ignore them sometimes becuase they…hurt? Sure we do. We stuff them away deep inside

ourselves. Do we stuff ourselves with food to push our emotions away?
Sure we do.

Frustration, such as running out of gas or losing your keys, finally
becomes so frustrating that it's too much to bear the pain of continuing
with the same old habits. We finally keep a fulltank or we get a big key
ring and hang the keys on a special hook!

You know only too well how frustrating it has been in the past to try
to lose weight, lose a pound or two and then gain them back. That
became so frustrating that it caused you to pick up this book, right?
This emotion finally stimulates a change as well. Our pot boils and boils
until we go to the stove, pour the tea, and drink it.

Confusion is so disturbing that you will do almost anything to get
out of it, and the interesting thing about this state is that the state of
confusion is when you are learning the most. Your brain is sorting
frantically for answers to get you back on track, and this is when most
of the "Ahas" come to force you in a new direction and get you out of
the pain. An *Aha* is when you receive a learning or an inspiration
within yourself.

Disappointment is the emotion that can cause you to say: "I give up"
and for this particular emotion it is the most important to ask questions
like: "What were my expectations in this situation?", "How can I change
*my own thinking* to alter the outcome?" and "What can I learn from
this?". The last thing you want to do is disappoint yourself.

Once you have changed your state and your attitude you can feel the
relief and aknowledge in your mind your new state of feeling and being.
Take time to observe your attempt to change, and allow the feelings of
that success. Small steps count!

For example here are some of the statements that keep me going forward when I say them aloud.

I am relentless toward reaching my goal

I have run out of ways to sabotage myself

I'm responsible for my world, my feelings and my outcome

I am flowing in motion

I am light hearted

"Where there's a will there's a way"

Life is what I make it

If I change my life I can change my behavior

There is always a way I'm committed to me

I have the power within myself to be healthy and happy in all that I do

All behavior is either an act of love or a cry for help

I'm a visionary in action, transcending my history of thinking…and I am relentless in my taking action for myself.

One of my favorite emotions is curiosity. When I begin to ask myself questions, it can be like coming out of a maze of emotions like fear, shame and anxiety. The minute I become curious about an event or circumstance and ask questions I throw yourself into a new state of curiosity and therefore on the path to finding a solution to almost any question. I begin to feel a new sense of direction. More questions lead me to more answers.

Try it now with one of your statements about a negative emotion. How about: "I feel depressed because I'm so overweight". Now go throught the questionsabove. Then write down the emotions you are having and go ahead and feel them and then ask yourself the questions that apply to your situation.

Do you find yourself in a curiosity state? If not, stay confused until you do. This exercise will take some time because you will enjoy the change and feel your own power. You will pop out of confusion into curiosity.

And now... your new body...really feel it, visualize it, color it, dress it, whatever you can do to imagine it...and once again observe your possibilities. You can begin to feel more lighthearted now as you make up your own affirmations such as: "I'm on my way to being myself!", "This time I'm not going to disappoint myself!", "I'm a possibility in action!".

This is my favorite: "*I'm a visionary in action and I am relentlessly and actively transcending my history!*"

"I no longer allow myself to be heavy in mind or body"

"I am letting go of the possibility of being overweight"

Now, ask yourself this question and give an honest answer: "How do I feel when I focus on being overweight?". And now: "How do I feel when I change my focus and my emotions to being my ideal weight?"

The only way to notice the difference is to feel it and respond to yourself with honesty...and of course...love and self respect.

# Chapter 10

## Love and the Lightness of Being

All of us have received at one time or another conditional love, instead of unconditional love we have all heard hidden messages "When you do well in school, I'll love you", "When you live up to my standards, I'll love you" or "When you clean your plate, I'll love you", "When you become perfect by doing things my way, I'll love you". From these messages we can also learn to accept ourselves only on a conditional basis, such as when we are **good** in the eyes of others.

In my seminars I have noticed that what participants want to take home from the learnings the most is *self acceptance*. They want a comfortable feeling in their bodies, a feeling of well being. I truly believe what that means, is we all want and need to be loved just for being who we are, not for what we do and how we do it. When we experience a loving relationship and it is fulfilling, we share unconditional love and are accepted by our loved ones. What that ultimately means is that we are free to make mistakes and learn from them, without being shamed or blamed for having a different view of situations and circumstances. Conditional love on the other hand can create in one a feeling of unworthiness for being yourself, and only through attempting to please the partner can one be accepted. When this occurs, we can become aware of the possibility of reaching into the

69

refrigerator to fill an empty feeling of not being accepted. What are our empty feelings about? Could it be we are feeling unlovable?

So what does love have to do with losing weight? When misunderstandings arise in loving relationships, as they inevitably do from time to time, a fear of loss can occur. If loss is not apparent, the criticizing and blaming can leave a feeling of emptiness temporarily or on a permanent basis. How these thoughts and fears connect with losing weight is what I call filling the emptiness *within* with food instead of love or a replacement for acceptance and satisfaction with one's self.

Conditional love, on the other hand, can create in one a feeling of unworthiness, and only through attempting to try and please the others can one be accepted. When you are facing the thought of not being accepted, why not take a time out just for yourself? Give yourself a chance to ask and you shall receive. What am I feeling? Am I feeling unlovable?

We have learned in previous chapters that in order to receive or get love, a child learns to please the parents. There are many families who give and receive love freely. I speak from a point of view where love is conditional, or in cases of families where there is conflict, and as a result love is withheld for various reasons or a parent doesn't know how to simply say "I love you".

When love is withheld, or not freely given, the notion of being unlovable can arise, and the result can be *discomfort* expressed in the form of frustration, depression, or even less self trust about what the future may bring. Food has the potential of filling the emptiness immediately (the quick fix), and it is sometimes associated with immediate comfort as well, as in the past. We all want love and need love and sometimes we will even accept the illusion of love or a love substitute in our desperation of trying to fill our empty hearts.

We could spend years trying to earn the love we deserve from all those around us, or we can change the way we think about our own self acceptance. So far we find that, there are no limits to our human potential. As we learn and grow the possibility of our own potential also becomes greater. When we accept ourselves unconditionally we become free to offer all that we have learned to others, to give love to others and to give love to ourselves.

Beware now of the idea of giving and receiving love. When we give love and receive love from one other person the emptiness is instantly gone. Think about a loving situation or conversation you have shared either recently or in the past. This could be with a friend or your partner. Just notice if you had an empty feeling. Take a moment now to reflect. Remember a time when you were totally involved with this other person. All of your attention was immersed in the loving feelings. You can see the person in your imagination and even refeel the loving feelings. As you go back in your mind, you will once again have the same feelings, and just allow them to be again in your imagination and in your whole body. When you are giving and receiving love, it's just not possible to be occupied with feelings of emptiness, is it? Stay with this now, as an awareness with yourself. Put yourself into this blissful state so that it becomes real for you. As you reflect on this beautiful state of love in this way you can realize that love is all around you. You don't have to try to go and find it to receive it. It is within you.

A client, Alex, came to me one day feeling very distraught. His story has value in relating to you the significance of being in a loving situation. Alex said to me: "Last night I looked in the mirror as you told me to do and I began to notice, while looking at myself, all the loving attributes about myself. I became very honest with myself and told myself in the mirror *you are really a good person Alex!* I noticed when I told myself that feedback my face began to soften, and I even smiled at myself knowing that I believed it. I told myself: *I am always doing the best I can and my intention is to enjoy my life and share with others in a loving way.* It was a profound experience for me, in that I couldn't feel bad about myself when I was feeling so loving *to me.* I felt complete and full. This morning I went to the beach for a walk. *I remembered looking in the mirror* and once again felt a surge of power within myself as I also felt the power of the universe by the sea. The same loving feelings came back. Then it seemed they were gone again and I had a feeling of powerlessness. I tried to get my power back but it just didn't seem to return. Where did my power go?".

I told him to just go through the day speaking with others and sharing his experience and to be willing to trust that his power would come back. He looked at me discouraged because I didn't seem to have the direct answer he was looking for. A few hours later he returned full of excitement and I said: "What happened?". He said: "Beat came up to me and he was so discouraged with himself that he was going to go home, he was going to give up on himself because he was feeling depressed. I told Beat: *"Oh Beat don't go home now, for perhaps there is something you can learn by staying. You have nothing to lose by staying, I'll be here with you, I'm working hard on myself and it feels very painful to be making changes too. Just sit here with me and we'll go through this learning together. Perhaps we won't be sorry when you stay, but you could regret leaving if you go".*

Beat looked at Alex and said: "You think so? Well OK, I'll stay". Alex said: "I don't know what happened but all of a sudden I felt this surge of power within myself again". I said: "That's it Alex, you got it. Every time you give your power in the form of love to another human being it comes back in the form of personal power, doesn't it? You told yourself you are basically good and what makes you powerful is to share all that is love about yourself with others, right? And the minute you do it, it comes back to you, like your own reflection in the mirror! And the power and the love is always all around you. It's the way the universe works when we are in synchronicity with ourselves. You know now you will never lose your power and if it temporarily appears that it is gone, it will show up again sometimes in the most surprising and delightful ways. Trust it, try it, play with it, enjoy it, and the more you learn about yourself the more confident you become and the more it comes back to you!".

What if you were to believe in the best of all you are? And what if while you are becoming the best of all you are already, you give the best of yourself to others? I truly believe you wouldn't have to rely on food to become fulfilled, because all the love you need will come back to you from the most surprising people in the most surprising ways.

In *Love is letting go of fear* I read: "Love remains constant, only the particular person from whom we come to expect it may change. Nothing can interfere with the promise of comfort and love except our interpretation, and that will always interfere because it will cause us to look dishonestly at where we are and what surrounds us. This instant we have everything we need. Within this instant we have everything the key word is within. We can therefore trust what happens because there will never be a time when it will not be NOW".

When we shame and blame and judge or we are shamed, blamed and judged by others, we block the loving emotions that are our intention with others in sharing and giving and receiving love. We have love all around us, but this love cannot be experienced if we are focusing our minds on everything except what is at hand that is loving. We can not experience love and fear at the same time. We can tune our mental T.V. to only one channel at a time, or we only have static on an empty screen.

When being loving person in a love relationship means we are in pain, we are in danger of losing our own self value. And when we lose our own sense of self value, we can feel crazy sometimes and obsessive in relation to food.

When being in love means we are trying to fix our loved one or make excuses for their behavior, we are becoming perhaps addicted or obsessed with the object of our love instead of just giving love freely.

When we try to give more love while being blamed, and when we are involved in a relationship that includes alcohol and other drugs, our own response to overeating can be easily triggered, even when we are not aware of it. Our unconscious always protects us and if food gives us a boundary of protection we will eat to be protected. Sometimes we block ourselves so as to not allow our boundaries to be violated. Love itself can become an addiction in that in dysfunctional relationships one has a belief that self sacrifice the way to get love. This wall of protection through over eating and becoming overweight gives a feeling of shuting out unloving criticism as may have been the case in one's past history. When we love obsessively and eat obsessively we are really operating out of fear, fear of being alone and fear of being unloveable and unworthy of love. We fear and believe we will be rejected or abandoned.

I realize now that when I was between 16 and 20 years old I had eaten to fill the emptiness of not receiving love from my father. My mother was also very much needing love and the two of us together fed ourselves to find the feeling of fullness. My father just didn't know how to express his love because his mother abandoned him, and he literally took himself to a boarding home and raised himself. My mother was raised the youngest of 11 children and her father died at her age of 2.

From then on, she grew up with an abusive stepfather. Her eating and becoming fat offered her a wall of protection against her stepfather's sexual inuendos, or so she thought.

My parents didn't want any children. So I turned out to be an accident, and delivered to 2 people who simply hadn't learned how to express love. Eating was a time I could get fulfillment...or so I thought.

I can only imagine this may trigger thoughts about your own childhood if it does remember. First comes the awareness of how we have become the persons we are.

Transformations come in glimpses so small we can miss them every day. I wonder how many we miss. Each time we have an idea or a thought we have the opportunity for learning about ourselves and acting on that opportunity.

I wonder how curious we must become or how uncomfortable before we pay attention, before we listen, before we watch, before we feel we are really transforming to the only fulfilling message there is. I believe the message of self acceptance and self love that is unconditional is simply to be aware of the message of love. Am I in love or am I in fear? Ask your heart.

I really think this is the way we ultimately fill our emptiness. All the food we eat, that gives the illusion of our need of fullness being met, only results in our feeling less accepted by ourselves.

Today I choose to give my love freely.

At age 16 I noticed I was different because of being fat. I had many girl friends, but no boy friends. I felt the pain when at the beach in the summertime the boys played games of picking up the girls and throwing them in the water, and nobody picked me up, I was too heavy. I associated that to being unattractive and I believed if I did get the chance to have a date, it was only with the left overs, in other words, all the wonderful guys chose girls with good figures. I was starving for love and acceptance, so I ate because it was the only thing that came close to filling my emptiness. And I was looking for love. Love was all around me, but I didn't know it, and my interpretation, my meaning, caused me to believe that I was unloveable.

And we have already realized what happens when we have a limiting belief. We settle for what we believe because we don't think we deserve more.

I thought love was conditional on my being slim, therefore I learned also not to give love openly because that contributed to a fear I would either lose the love because I was fat, or I would be rejected because of my size. Years later when I was finally in an environment where I was respected and loved just for being me, I could let go of all my extra weight and still feel fulfilled and lovable.

As I learned, so I transfer my learning to you with pleasure and gratitude for this opportunity. I am also recycling my old self.

I wish you the capability to freely accept love from others because of your deep down convinction that you are lovable just the way you are. Being worthwhile and deserving of all the love around you makes it far easier to feel empathy and compassion for others and to cast out self doubt and replace it with self love.

# Chapter 11

## Planning

You are determined to lose weight now and you have made the decision to give yourself the power from within to go ahead, to take action in reaching your desired goal of becoming, exactly the lifestyle you will enjoy. Planning the next step, will allow all your creativity in planning to be a path for you to follow every day. Along with creatively deciding what to eat every day we, who are compulsive in our food habits, can make also an **emotional plan** so that strength from our very soul, our inner self emits from us each day.

Morning can be your time for you to make your plan. For some of you, this creative time for yourself can occur the first thing in the morning, and it can be a luxurious time while you are still cozy in your bed. You will find that your intended state is as important to plan as what you are going to eat, and here in these quiet moments you can find *within yourself* all the love and carefree thoughts to carry you through one day at a time. Just be in the present, with no thoughts of inability or failure because you have learned it is possible for you to direct your possibilities through change. You are committed to your purpose of fulfilling your own desires and dreams of a totally healthy body. Your own self direction is the person you really are within. If others of you find the evening a better time to make your daily plan, then by all means do this in the evening, for you understand your own time clock inside. When you are free within yourself without worrying about the past, you can feel your full energy to intend and give attention to what it is that you want and deserve for yourself.

The eating part is very easy to follow, as you can choose from a variety of healthy energizing foods. There is no strict plan for measuring the right proportions of certain kinds of foods, so you never have to worry that you will not eat the right food to carry you through your weight loss program. Here we will concentrate only on a variety of foods that are enhancing your desired weight loss.

Lowering your fat intake in your diet is a great start! It's possible you haven't even thought of foods where fat is included in amounts not necessary for your daily consumption. This fat can occur in such foods as french fries or any fried foods, rich salad dressings and sauces used to be placed on top of meats and vegetables. Usually these sauces are oozing with butter or oil and the truth about too many fats and oils is, they can also turn to fat in the body.

Substitute another methods of cooking, such as broiling or grilling without the use of fat and oils. Purchase only lean meat and you begin already to cut the amount of calories and fat consumption way down. These little secrets just make your plan easy to follow while creating your own desired results.

Now we have mentioned what to eliminate from your daily food intake, and now let's get down to all the wonderful foods you can have in unlimited amounts for your enjoyment. No longer do you have to suffer by trying to eat less and starve yourself! Let's brain storm all your possibilities for daily healthy enjoyable eating.

Why not begin your day with fruit and whole grains, and that means always have a big bowl of various kinds of fruit available to you. Having to run to the store could cause you to grab anything nearest you to satisfy a moment of hunger, and reaching for a piece of fruit, whatever if appealing to you, will give you a nutricious start in your day and keep you on track. You simply will not reach out for donuts, because you will think about it first, and instantly remember ...oops...these three donuts are just an old habit, from perhaps many years, and say to yourself: "Today I am eating only the foods that are keeping me on track in becoming slim", smile to yourself and then move on take a rich corn bread or a whole wheat.

I have heard some people say: "Everything that is good, I can't have". When you are aware of these old habits that contributed to your overweight condition you can smile to yourself acknowledging to yourself that you are changing old habits, old beliefs and are replacing them with new knowledge and a new understanding about yourself. You are taking action for you.

For breakfast add a piece of cheese (lite), a beverage of your choice such as coffee or tea, as these beverages do not add to your calories intake. Of course lots of water flushes your system and water based foods, such as fruits and vegetables, will never cause you to gain weight, but rather will flush through your system and give you all the enjoyment of satisfying your hunger.

It is a real advantage to be able to purchase lite cheese, lite jogurt and skim milk. You may say to yourself at first: "Why do I have to give up something?". If you find yourself beginning to feel sorry for yourself, stop, think about what you are thinking and remember *what you want.* Just know you are simply reframing your thinking, and that allows you to go forward, change old attitudes about how hard it is to change, because that is only your old way of thinking. You are really committed to reaching your goal, you can at any time review one of the previous chapters to get you back into your own way of taking action. You can do this when you take each day as I step forward. And of course don't forget to enjoy all the feelings of your success each day. "I can do this and I am doing this". Small steps count.

If you want a piece of bread for breakfast, go ahead and have it, have 2 pieces if you like, for what is most important for you is to be comfortable with yourself while you are losing weight.

The mid day meal can be full of a variety of salads and vegetables complete with a variety of whatever of these you like. I do not suggest you have a bowl of spinach if you don't like it because it just wouldn't give you pleasure, and this program is not about giving yourself any pain, right? If you enjoy meat or fish in the mid day, by all means, have it. If you enjoy bread, have a piece, or even better 2 pieces, all the while considering what is important to you in this daily plan. What do you really want? To lose all the weight you desire, right? Bread will not make you fat! Eat with pleasure!

In the evening repeat the same menu as you had for the mid day meal if you are very hungry. Take 4 or 5 fruits and vegetables, 4 or 5 fruits and 3 handfuls carbohydates for the day.

First ask yourself: "How hungry am I?" or "What do I really need?". If it's a bowl of fruit and that's it, great. If you want a huge salad from an available salad bar, where you don't have to prepare it all yourself, then treat yourself, only remembering to be aware of the fat content, and or sugar in prepared foods. Canned fruits contain large amounts of sugar, and when you can order fresh fruit, it is of course to your advantage. Anywhere you can cut the fat or sugar, you win! 3 big handfuls of carbohydrates per day will go right through your body without causing you to gain weight.

If you have the urge to eat something late in the evening don't deny yourself because you are telling yourself food is something you really need to satisfy your hunger. Try a banana or an apple, eat it slowly and really enjoy it, and chances are that's enough to satisfy you. Drink a nice warm tea, one that you really enjoy and then go to bed, feeling very satisfied about You. Be willing to try something new! You don't really need that big ham and cheese sandwich before you go to bed!

In your planning time you are also going to be aware of who you are inside for mastering your pick and choose according to your needs for this day, asking yourself:"What do I need today?".

**Courage**—Go inside yourself and find your courage to change old habits in the present. You can't change the fact that you have become overweight, but you can change your actions. Making these changes requires the *courage* for you to start out on a new and unknown path. Courage means you are taking action inspite of sometimes being afraid. It takes courage to say "No" to extra portions of food that are no longer necessary, and to do it in such a way that you feel good about yourself. It takes courage to live with the truth instead of living with old comfortable illusions. Sometimes it takes courage to step out in a new direction because old fears, like old habits, can creep back into our lives...

**Changing mistakes into learning opportunities**—Dwelling on what we haven't done in the past is a waste of time and gets us nowhere. Allow yourself to benefit from all you have learned from the past. If a particular attitude from the past stands in your way of staying on your plan and you are feeling guilty, at any time *that old attitude about a past action can be changed*! It just indicates that taking 5 steps forward and 3 steps back doesn't just happen by accident! You have not yet learned what you need to know about yourself in a certain way. Being aware of the circumstances that make you vulnerable to overeating prepares you to be ready for temptation, and if there are certain foods that in the past you could not resist, then just don't have those foods available. Emotional food binging let's us now that we are not living in a way that satisfies our basic needs. Go inside yourself and say: "Let me learn from my past today. I can change what no longer works for me". My *guilt feelings* no longer need to cause me to reach out for food. My feelings are not about hunger for food! My feelings are about something else. Go back to your heart and ask: "What's going on? What am I feeling? What does that mean?" "AHA!"

**Movement**—When it comes to overeating we are either getting better at resolving and changing our habits or we are staying stuck. And sometimes we are even moving backwards. Live in the now not looking back on the illusion that there was much pleasure gained by eating a lot of food. Now instead, a small amount of intension can become a large amount. Instead of pleasure from overeating you will begin to transcend those feelings of remembered pain. When you are making progress you will be *motivated* to go forward. If you should notice you are taking a step backwards, just observe that, and be honest with yourself. Ask yourself what you really need to give you emotional satisfaction. Be aware of constantly making excuses in the past. With your new awareness you can turn around and start going forward again. Do it today. Small steps count!

**Illusions**—Those of us who have struggled with our weight, have lived in an illusion that a certain sugar or starch will temporarily satisfy a painful moment, and later learned we gained more pain than pleasure from this illusion. Practicing honesty with yourself today will cause you to be able to separate illusion of pleasure about overeating with the reality that you can face yourself in the mirror letting go of past illusions, and simply saying to yourself: "I know much more now about me, and today I am taking responsibility for my actions, and therefore, my reality".

**Conserving energy for what is not important today**—In your plan you need all the energy available to you from deep within. Sometimes you may need an extra hour of sleep that will enable you to be well rested and not crabby or feeling stress. Overactivity can contribute to overeating in that it can be too easy to reach for the foods that are not helpful in your plan. Sometimes when we are tired we are less able to resist temptation. In your plan today create a balance of not doing unnecessary things that you can do tomorrow. Conserve your energy, pace your time, and make your day *for you*. Sometimes this means saying no to activities which take your energy unnecessarily. Only you can best decide to use the strength and energy you have to make your day totally enjoyable and keep you on track. Conserve your energy today. If you need more sleep, give it to yourself. It could be that one more hour of sleep can give you all the energy you need to cause you to keep on keeping on. Do you need a time just for you today? Oh, it is so important to take that time for yourself. You are important!

**Responding to old messages**—We all have the choice of replaying old messages that have transpired in our lives whether they are positive or negative. Some of our old tapes are negative and self destructive with resentments and fears. When one of these old tapes begin to play we may find ourselves going to the refrigerator to satisfy that old pain. You can begin this day to take a mental dry cleaning of any discomfort, like beating yourself for making mistakes in the past or for saying something you wish you wouldn't have said. Often there is a guilty feeling. You never have the intention of hurting another person, and you know your mistakes or setbacks are only opportunities for learning. Simply stop today and be grateful for all you have learned about all that is good and resourceful about yourself, and then allow the feelings of self love and love for others just record over the old messages, giving you a warm understanding of yourself. You can purify your own thoughts and feelings today. We, as humans, have the gifts of choice. Choose for yourself the freedom to reach what you really want.

**Risk of rejection**—Reaching out to others can feel like taking a risk. Exposing your needs dissolves your facade of self sufficiency. Being vulnerable exposes yourself to the world and has in the past been very frightening because it opens the doors for others to begin shaming or blaming you. Each day as you open up to others and show yourself just who you are, you will see your own mirror image in others. Today as you allow yourself to be you, enjoy seeing the mirror image of your new self in the eyes of others. Notice your own fulfillment in their responses. Don't forget to notice and realize how beautiful you already are.

**Physical Action**—Each day as you plan how your body will exercise, create an exercise for yourself that is enjoyable to you. Don't force yourself to run 10 miles or something that you dread. What is important is keeping your heart rate up for at least 40 minutes each time you exercise. Even more important than that is being honest with yourself about how much you exercise. If you say: "Oh I walk a lot every day, so that's good enough". That really is good enough. These days of a variety of courses offer the enjoyable exercise for you. You don't have to jump up and down in an aerobics class for 20 year olds if you are 55, you don't even have to do that if you are 20. In every area where you live you can now find the exercise suitable to your pleasure. If you are fortunate enough to live in a beautiful place of nature, you can learn how exilarating it can be to walk briskly for an hour or so.

If you absolutely don't want to exercise for 30 minutes or an hour, do it for 20 minutes. Regularity is important, so it has to be an exercise you enjoy or you will quit! Me too! Small steps count big time!

# Chapter 12

## Role Modeling

Have you ever wondered why some people are so successful, and others are not? And have you ever wondered about the difference in the way human beings respond to what happens to them?

Why do some persons overcome all the disasters and complications in life and triumph, while others who have many advantages seem to turn their lives into problem states and misery?

*I believe it is because those who succeed know they have choices to change the meaning of life circumstances to learning opportunities.*

The way we communicate with ourselves predicts our enjoyment and our responses to life's situations. Our response ability leads to success in our life. In every area of your life that you want to change and make an opportunity for yourself, there is a person or many persons who are already experts. The example that is relevant here is, you can invest time and study into modeling persons who are successful at remaining slim and healthy and you can produce the same result. Learning what they eat, how they eat, what they think about their bodies and what their beliefs are, can contribute to your own knowledge of how to reach your desired weight and keep it. When I discovered this wonderful short cut, I looked around and found several persons I admired as having been successful in what I needed to know about becoming slim and healthy. There have been persons in my life who knew all about how to meet their specific goals much better than I, and I began to study those persons who overcame all obstacles in their way to get what they wanted. "If they can do it, I can too! And I really want to!".

In my personal life I realized in order to meet my goals of total health and fitness, I had to have a maximum amount of energy, and be congruent in what I was teaching, which paradoxically was how to lose weight. I had to be a living example of all I knew was true for me. I set my outcome of a radiantly energetic illuminating example of being exactly what I teach. I even imagined myself on "Good Morning America" or CNN the same as my role model Barbara Walters and every morning as I watched her, I learned her skills of poise and gracefullness with a dynamic speaking ability. I pretended I was Barbara Walters, and made a role play with myself, as if I were the one who was interviewing famous persons from around the world, and showing women and men how to reach their goals.

At that time, Jane Fonda was an expert in health and fitness. She weighed about the same as I imagined myself to be, and she and I are about the same age.

I decided if she could be slim and healthy and train others to do the same that I could do it too...if I focused on it, decided what I wanted and believed in my own ability to take action. The first thing I did was buy her fitness video and her programs on fitness on cassettes to listen in the car. Then I studied them to the point where I associated myself with everything she did. I also joined an aerobics class an began to study the methods, so that I knew the routines so well I could teach it myself. I went to several classes to observe until I found the right one. I learned what all the experts were advising that was just suited to my needs, because I wanted to have fun and be comfortable with myself or I would give up. I know that! I didn't want to pound my bones on a wooden floor and jump around making myself exhausted. I also read everything I could find on Jane. I even wrote her a letter and invited her to open my future imagined weight loss retreat center. I've never mailed it, but I sure had fun writing it. And even if I didn't mail it, it began to process in my mind my own possibilities. I played it out in my mind as if I was really doing it just like her.

Then I began to take action eating and drinking nutrutious low calorie foods that I liked, and comitted myself to one hour of aerobics 3 times per week. If for some reason I couldn't get to the aerobics studio, I would substitute one hour of fast walking wherever I was...so that there were no excuses like I don't have time, or I'm too tired. And in the aerobics class I stood in the front row, where I could see in a wall to wall mirror, all my fat jumping and bulging. Over the next weeks and months I watched it melting away! That gave so much pleasure to me, doing something just for me.

While you are reading this, begin to think also of people you know that you can model. Who does what you want...better than you?

For tenacity and motivation, I modeled a 72 year old man who was in tip top fitness condition. One day I said to him: "Gene, how do you stay so fit, and where do you get the motivation to exercise?". He gave me the answer in one simple sentence: "*Mary, keeping fit is number one in my life*". I used that sentence each morning when I woke up, until it became a part of me. In this way I made him a role model for my own practice.

Then I began to notice many slim women at the studio, on the streets and in shopping centers, and I saw that some women were very graceful and others were various stages from regal to sloppy looking, and as I began to think about how I looked when I moved, I asked myself, who were the beautiful thin and graceful women in the world. One, I decided was Meryl Streep, and the other who seemed to have it all, and charisma too, was Tina Turner, who is also my age. I took myself to a concert in Basel to observe her. The repertoire she had with 80'000 persons complete with graceful movement and fun loving confidence was incredible. I was moved by her energy and charisma. And I found myself later pretending I was giving seminars with Tina. I had so much fun playing those roles. It was energy giving to continue going toward my goal of 130 pounds, because with role modeling it was a pleasure. I played the role of all the parts I was becoming: Tina, Jane and Gene.

And still there was another person who was managing fitness better than I, my colleague and good friend, Ed Charlesworth. He was a marathon runner and my partner in "Inner Thin" groups in Texas, and he not only practiced his program of weight loss and fitness with excercising every day, but he invited his client to join him every day for bicycling, walking, running and eating out at restaurants ordering sandwiches with vegetables and no mayonaise, and visiting the local grocery stores to get an education about what was available in lite foods. So I did the same, and started my own aerobics classes, went shopping for aerobics clothes with clients who thought they were too fat for jogging suits, and we *walked* during the hour of weight loss instructions, instead of sitting at the table!

I can only imagine you are already beginning to think about persons in your life or even someone you have noticed, read about or seen on TV that you admire as experts in their fields of interest. From using my example, give yourself the opportunity now to play this role modeling game. Always, first think again about your intension. Then spend some time thinking and imagining others who have conquered the battle of the bulge, and begin to study just how they have taken action toward their accomplishments. Let's make a graph. I do it like this.....

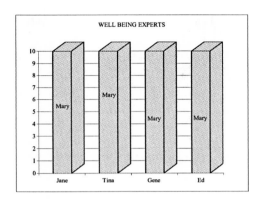

It's a simple bar graph. I give a simple grade of excellence from 1 to 10 as the highest achievement of excellence. I of course gave all of my role models a grade of 10. Then I give myself a grade. Each week I notice my improvement and raised my grade. I must be really honest with myself because if I should not begin taking action in a weekly time space, I must acknowledge that too. When I can see it written on my graph, I learn from myself what I have left out and what I need to work on the most. Then I must do it because of being *comitted* and *responsible* to myself only, to reach my goal.

Ask yourself: "What do I need to enable myself more easily to reach my goal? Do I need courage, confidence, trust in myself, support from others?". Then realize who it is that can give that to you. Maybe what you really need is love, unconditional love, just for being you, and encouragement to continue toward your goal. Maybe you need someone to tell you how good you are doing. You could use a few confirmations about you. I once said to my husband: "I need your love, and then it's like I can climb mountains to reach anything I want!".

# Chapter 13

## *Your State of Excellence*

When you visualize your ideal weight in a meditative state you can feel delighted even excited just about thinking of the possibility. We have discussed thought, imagination, decision making and love, as it related to creating for ourselves our direction for fulfillment. This learning experience is only something we can cultivate through experience, in other words step by step. Your experience can be like stepping into a new pair of shoes that you have just purchased. You just love them because they look good! Now the first few days in the new shoes…and they might pinch a little. Perhaps they just don't feel as comfortable as the old worn out shoes. But do you throw them away because they pinch? No way! You keep on breaking them in…getting them to match better to your feet. In a few days the stiffness begins to relax and so do your feet. You begin to enjoy them. Only then are you willing to give the old ones up! Step by step, right?

To allign ourselves with a attitude of feeling good, we can allign our thoughts with appreciation of our small steps. "Today I am one step closer to my goal. Today I am in the new shoes". Your experience wil be confirmed. I can do this *today*.

Seek and you will find! And we are *all* seeking! Seeking and finding is something we do constantly. And not only once, every week or every

New Year's resolution…but every day. If you are sometimes down and enmeshed in self pity about how bad the world is…STOP, and ask yourself these questions:

1. How can I find and have what I am seeking?
2. How do I want to end this day today?

Think of a time when you got something you wanted. It could be a car, or a new pair of shoes that you really wanted, and you had to give some effort to get. Notice what happened to your attitude and your state of motivation. If you really *wanted* that pair of shoes, you could be out of money, tired from a long day's work, or in the middle of a snow storm, yet the *desire* and the *challenge* to do whatever it takes, propeled you to venture out, find the money, dress up warm, and go get those shoes! The point is, we create an adventure and a motivation to find what gives us pleasure. Notice, we never worry about our self confidence when seeking the pair of shoes we saw in the window, and just *must have*. And we find ourselves delighted when those shoes are properly placed in a sack, the transaction is completed, and we walk out of the store.

What we are looking for is our **desired state**. And what is a desired state? It's simply a state of pleasure! We are not seeking problem states that's for sure, even though we do find ourselves in undesirable states from time to time.

There is always a meaningful intention behind a desired state. In the shoe adventure, perhaps you want a certain pair of shoes to wear for a special evening…or perhaps this pair of shoes is attempting to give you a new image, and this is just one little step to reaching your state of being a "new you". Even if it is a pair of shoes to keep you warm for the winter, you are going in a direction to feel pleasure. This step counts. It's the beginning of getting what you want. It is remembering your intension with attention.

And just as the desired shoes are not going to magically appear on your doorstep, neither are you going to become automatically slim without taking action.

If you were to make a mental cookbook (like a road map) of your desired states so that you could feel good about your adventure of losing weight, what would be the necessary ingredients?

So here is your mental cookbook for achieving your desired state of being just how you want to be:

1 thought
2 or 3 visualizations of yourself as you want to be
1 bunch of words of encouragement
a dash of confidence
1 memory of past achievement
mixed with taking action vigorously until smooth and light

Combine all ingredients and exercise your ability to create effectively this fulfilling receipe.

Serve complete with candles as you become delighted.

Your nervous system cannot tell the difference between an imagined experience and a real experience. It reacts to what it imagines to be true". It is useful to realize that our bodies kinesthetically respond to every picture and sound we actually experience, remember experiencing, or imagine experiencing for example. If before skiing the moguls on a steep run, I construct a picture of flawless skiing, my body believes that I am that skillful, and it responds with excitement and readiness. Blood sugar is up, adrenalin flows, endorfins are high, throat relaxes, taking in more air, the liver produces more glucose, adding fuel to tissues, pupils dilate, sharpening visual perceptions, breathing is stimulated and all of this mental exercise creates in the body the response of flowing or moving freely.

Understanding mastering and gaining flexibility of mental strategies is the key to successful movement toward your desired goal. *The body absolutely responds to its mentally imagined state.*

The importance of creating for yourself the desired state of being slim and healthy takes place in your mind first, and as you exercise according to your plan three or four times per week whether it be walking, swimming or aerobics, your physical state in the process of taking action while exercising stimulates your total desired state while increasing your motivation.

Just remember, when you do this, there is only success for you. So why don't you go ahead and put yourself in your desired state now, exactly how you want to be and enjoy the process step by step.

# Chapter 14

## Spirituality

It is a pleasure to share with you my process and developments. Because I've been through similar problems and situations, I can reflect on how others feel, and can offer some solutions that have worked for me. An accumulated amount of experience and learning over the many years of my life have contributed to a wealth of understanding of the complicated multidimensional problems, solutions, and awakenings that can occur every day to us all. I also know it is important to acknowledge and give credit with deep respect to all persons with whom I come in contact as they pursue their heart's desires. Wherever they are on their journey in life. They deserve the highest regard. When I see that persons are being encouraged or helped because of my adding another piece to the puzzle of their lives I am often grateful to God, the Higher Power I consider always evident in this universe, my life, and the lives of others. I believe I am transfering and transcending grace and power from a higher source than myself to others. When problems surface, I notice sometimes I respond to daily activities in the same ways as those who come to me. Sometimes I wait until I am in pain before I ask for spiritual help and guidance, yet I know when I do ask for solutions, guidance, and direction, an answer always comes to me, even if the answer is a simple one. For example I'll get an insight, not necessarily a voice, but just a *knowing*. It will dawn on me, so to speak, to stop focusing on the problem I'm faced with, and focus rather on the solution; or something will say to me: "Practice what you say Mary, or listen to your inner self!".

Now where do these answers come from? I believe there is a force or source that is larger than myself, as if there is a purpose or a destiny toward which I am traveling through life. What I have noticed also, is that when I just let go of trying to make or demand or force my outcomes and dreams to happen, and allow them to unfold in their own time, whatever my present goal may be, a feeling of calmness or oneness with the universe comes over me. It is as if I can trust the very essence from which all my thoughts and goals are coming. When I have this calm understanding or knowing that I can trust the universe for literally everything, that I will in fact be given all the love I need, all the security and all the knowledge to pursue my own destiny, first of all my body relaxes and then my mind becomes clear to receive that which I want. I receive my gifts from God in order to recycle them and pass them on to others. *I am receiving the gifts I have been given to give.* When I try to force my goals to happen, and worry that I can't do something, or create a fear, such as an illusion of failure, I literally shut down, and stand in my own way. I become blocked.

I give you my own example here because for years, perhaps like some of you, I didn't know I could be really direct myself to becoming the slim and healthy person I desired.

I had some kind of an idea that I was destined to be fat. I tried every new diet that came out in books and quick fixes in magazines, and thought by some outside source I could master through others, calorie counting, or fasting, or eating only grapefruits and cucumbers to end my battle with weight. I finally found out I could place my thoughts and my desires into the universe, and be *willing to allow* them to happen, rather than to rely on other persons who were well meaning, to lose my weight for me. There is a difference in forcing or demanding your goal, and being willing to allow it to happen with faith and trust in yourself, and for this reason I add the notion of spirituality for enhancing your ideal weight loss.

Sometimes while I'm walking in the mountains looking at the beauty, hearing rushing streams, and feeling the earth under my feet as gravity pulls me down to the ground, all my senses seem to make me aware that everything around me is operating in perfect harmony with some kind of force or source that is larger than life as we know it and understand it. And even more, while in the beauty of nature, when I notice an army of ants, for example, all on a mission, with a purpose, all in line carrying food to a special place to function and survive, I can't help but wonder if all of us also have a purpose and a mission to carry a message, to transcend through certain stages in life in perfect harmony with everyone and everything else; a sort of evolving but with what I like to call a Higher Power or God.

This notion of a Higher Source or Power isn't the kind of thing you can measure or relate to facts; and none of us really know exactly what this spiritual power is, but all of us in our own way know that it exists. Philosophers for thousands of years have put labels on it, formed churches over it, and spent lifetimes trying to capture its essence. Many thousands of people in various religions have developed in their own way methods to harness their own spirituality. There seems to be comfort at all levels of understanding that we are not alone in this world, but rather are all bonded together by the idea or a belief in a Power larger than ourselves.

When we fall into the illusion of being powerless or out of control to master our own destinies, there seems to be a guiding influence, *when we acknowledge* it, that gives us knowledge of the right path to take in order to restore our balance and harmony. Some people call it an awakening or a vision. I am not trying to promote religion here, because for some of us, this larger than life experience can also be a hunch or an intuition, a thought or an idea, and it matters not where it comes from, except that it gives us the power to go forward, creating for ourselves a destiny that contributes *meaning* to our happiness and fulfillment.

Then our acceptance of ourselves, our destiny, and our desire to lose extra weight creates a willing atmosphere toward taking action.

Becoming slim and flexible can create a balance of energy and movement, breathing the fullness of life into our bodies with a light hearted emotion...or energy motion, enabling us to respond to ideas and thoughts from the universe and ask for help, while being willing to allow that resource in the universe, which is in harmony with all living beings, *to lead us to our destiny.* We can ask for courage, faith and motivation believing we can rely on our Higher Source. We can wonder and worry and obsess with a lot of extra food that is not harmonious with our body functions, or we can open the door to the knowledge of *our own resources,* whether that be within ourselves, or external in the universe allowing us to accept ourselves as harmonious with the very nature of life.

The importance of acknowledging a Higher Power is not to label it, or debate it, but rather consider it as having faith that all you desire is cause and effect or energy put into motion. It's as simple as planting a seed or seeds, with a trust you will also grow that which you planted.

When you believe that you are not alone and there is a Higher Power and if there are any such phenomena as miracles, they are produced through the state of mind known as faith.

Let's take the example of the power of faith as demonstrated by a man who was well known to all of civilization, Mahatma Gandhi of

India. In this man the world had one of the most outstanding examples known to civilization of the possibilities of faith. Gandhi had more power than any man living in his time, despite the fact that he had none of the tools of power, such as money, soldiers and guns of war. How did he come by that power? He created it out of his own understanding of faith, and through his ability to transplant that faith into the minds of two hundred million people. Gandhi influenced all these people to move in unison as a single mind. What other force on earth, except faith, could do as much? This is a perfect example that faith can transfer desire into its physical equivalent. It comes right down to faith in yourself and *your purpose,* and trust in your Higher Power as you understand it.

Napoleon Hill states in his book "Think and Grow Rich" that *faith* is the head chemist of the mind. When faith is blended with thought, the subconscious mind instantly picks up the vibration. Hill says that faith is a state of mind which may be induced, or created, by affirmation or repeated instructions to the subconscious mind through the principle of deep relaxation and meditation with a suggestion.

Consider your own purpose to lose weight. When you believe you will receive that for which you ask and that your subconscious will act on your belief, your subconscious passes it back to you in the form of faith followed by your definite plan to take action. Repetition of your positive thought to lose weight develops your own faith toward reaching your outcome.

When you dominate your mind by loving emotions you begin to give your unconscious messages and desires over and over as in your desire to lose weight, and through your practice, or your taking action every day, your faith in yourself also grows stronger and stronger. You begin to experience yourself as more harmonious, more power driven and motivated, and with a more trusting outlook on all that you endeavor to accomplish.

Each day, as you continue toward your goal of losing the exact amount of weight you desire, you can be willing to let go of the old beliefs about your overweight con- dition, as if you are shedding an old skin, like animals in nature, and transcending your past seasons from your wall of protection or emptiness to a new awareness of all that you are. Each day, as you have more faith and trust in yourself and your decision to lose weight, **allow** yourself to evolve into the healthy person you choose to be. You have **all the ressources in you.**

Give yourself appreciation for all that you know to be true and good about yourself. Allow your knowledge and new learning to flow through your body and your mind, like a river that never overflows its banks, but gently travels over rocks and reaches its destination in its own time, with faith and trust in your daily progress.

Experience every aspect of your life in different and more satisfying ways than when you relied on outdated habits, resources and old worn out thoughts  from the past that are no longer useful in your transformation. Unrestricted by limiting thoughts, attitudes and negative emotions, you can now enjoy a freer and more expansive life. As you let go of judging others, you lighten your own burdens, you can turn inward and each day be renewed with enthusiasm and joy, transforming your hearts desires to that of your own well being and satisfaction.

Regardless of the confusion and discord around all of us, our trust in a Higher Power in the universe keeps us serene and peaceful because we believe in a constant source of strength, assurance, and comfort. During times of uncertainty, practice each day at a time learning and experiencing the rewards of faith, realizing that any number of possibilities could delay in learning the outcome of a particular event. You can accept the reality of any situation as you carry out your daily activities. And most of all, **accept yourself,** just as you are, realizing you always have a positive intention in all that you do, deep within, and that you are progressing toward being the best of all that you already are.

# *About the Author*

Mary Bray, M.A. has dedicated her life to helping people from around the world reach their perfect weight. She received her psychological training at the University of Houston, Texas. Based in Switzerland since 1987, her books, programs and private consultations focus on the healing connections in mind, body and spirit.

0-595-14815-8